Hysteria

According to the medical world, hysteria is a thing of the past, an outdated diagnosis that has disappeared for good. This book argues that hysteria is in fact alive and well.

Hyperventilating, we rush from one incident into the next – there is hardly time for a breather. From the worldwide run on toilet paper to cope with coronavirus fears to the overheated discussions about immigration and overwrought reactions to the levels of crime and disorder around us, we live in a culture of hysteria. While hysteria is typically discussed in emotional terms – as an obstacle to be overcome – it nevertheless has very real consequences in everyday life. Irritating though this may be, hysteria needs to be taken seriously, for what it tells us about our society and way of life. That is why Marc Schuilenburg examines what hysteria is and why it is fuelled by a culture that not only abuses, but also encourages and rewards it.

Written in a clear and direct style, this book will appeal to students and scholars of sociology, criminology and philosophy, and all those interested in hysteria and how it permeates late modern society.

Marc Schuilenburg is Professor at the Faculty of Criminal Law and Criminology at VU University Amsterdam, the Netherlands. He is the author of *The Securitization of Society*.

'Schuilenburg's sociological analysis of hysteria gives us a powerful insight into the rise of reactionary right wing politics rooted in fear, anger, and frustration sweeping the US and much of the rest of the world. Their sense of power-lessness in the face of changing landscapes of power has been a major factor in the rise of punitive and authoritarian policing, mass incarceration, and the sca-pegoating of immigrants. But he also raises the possibility of a positive hysteria targeting economic inequality, climate change, and a cyclical politics of racism and xenophobia.'

Alex Vitale, author of *The End of Policing*

'In a work that crosses from the history of medicine to the rise of anti-immi-grant violence in Europe, Schuilenburg follows "hysteria" from the official catalogue of mental illnesses to a kind of cultural experience on a collective level. An astoundingly imaginative and keenly observed work of scholarship.'

Jonathan Simon, author of *Mass Incarceration on Trial: A Remarkable Court Decision and the Future of Prisons in America*

'Though fallen from fashion within psychology, in this important new volume Marc Schuilenburg makes a powerful case for the continued sociological rele-vance of *hysteria* to an understanding of our contemporary condition. Far from having disappeared it is everywhere and he details its manifestations in matters as widespread as the heated nature of our politics, our greedy and sometimes violent consumerism, through to what passes for interaction and debate in social media. In Schuilenburg's hands *hysteria* becomes an important tool in the sociological diagnosis of our current ills and our future possibilities.'

Tim Newburn, author of *Criminology*

'Marc Schuilenburg offers a calm, critical and deeply considered analysis of hysteria and its sometimes hysterical history.'

Jeff Ferrell, author of *Drift: Illicit Mobility and Uncertain Knowledge*

'An eye opener, for those who want to escape the hustle and bustle of everyday life.'

Paul Verhaeghe, author of *What About Me? The Struggle for Identity in a Market-Based Society*

'Suffused with fear, uncertainty and panic, the state of world is no laughing matter. In his new book, Marc Schuilenburg resuscitates a term once disregarded as imprecise and hyperbolic, giving us a language to understand and describe our frantic present, proving himself again to be one of the most creative, indeed pres-cient critics of crime, media and politics writing today.'

Travis Linnemann, author of *Media and Crime in the U.S.*

Hysteria

Crime, Media, and Politics

Marc Schuilenburg

Translated by
Vivien D. Glass

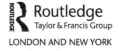
Routledge
Taylor & Francis Group

LONDON AND NEW YORK

First published 2021
by Routledge
2 Park Square, Milton Park, Abingdon, Oxon OX14 4RN

and by Routledge
52 Vanderbilt Avenue, New York, NY 10017

Routledge is an imprint of the Taylor & Francis Group, an informa business

© 2021 Marc Schuilenburg

Translated by Vivien D. Glass

Published in Dutch by Boom Filosofie 2019

British Library Cataloguing-in-Publication Data
A catalogue record for this book is available from the British Library

Library of Congress Cataloging-in-Publication Data
Names: Schuilenburg, Marc, 1971- author.
Title: Hysteria : crime, media, and politics / Marc Schuilenburg ; translated by Vivien D. Glass.
Description: Milton Park, Abingdon, Oxon ; New York, NY : Routledge, 2021. | Includes bibliographical references and index. |
Identifiers: LCCN 2020044779 | ISBN 9780367473464 (hardback) | ISBN 9780367473488 (paperback) | ISBN 9781003035022 (ebook)
Subjects: LCSH: Hysteria–History.
Classification: LCC RC532 .S36 2021 | DDC 616.85/24–dc23
LC record available at https://lccn.loc.gov/2020044779

ISBN: 978-0-367-47346-4 (hbk)
ISBN: 978-0-367-47348-8 (pbk)
ISBN: 978-1-003-03502-2 (ebk)

Typeset in Bembo
by Taylor & Francis Books

This publication has been made possible with financial support from the Dutch Foundation for Literature and the Koningsheide Foundation.

Contents

Foreword

Jeff Ferrell

In this book Marc Schuilenburg offers a calm, critical and deeply considered analysis of hysteria and its sometimes hysterical history. Early in that history, as Schuilenburg shows, hysteria came to life as a thoroughly gendered phenomenon, allegedly the product of wombs wandering insatiably inside women's bodies and of witches working in league with the devil. By the late 19th century the prominent French physician Jean-Martin Charcot had resituated hysteria as a phenomenon of physiology and heredity – and by theatrically performing his findings before crowds that included the likes of William James and Sigmund Freud, he had popularised his analysis to the point that, not surprisingly, diagnoses of hysteria proliferated.[1] Freud himself next relocated hysteria, this time into the realm of the subconscious and the purview of psychoanalysis. Later, Foucault would move hysteria once again, via a critique that positioned it as a biosocial issue tied to discipline and regulation.

Freud's contribution, as Schuilenburg explains, was to understand hysteria as 'a medium for communicating a message that, for a host of reasons, could not be conveyed in any other way'. For Freud, this referred to an individual's repressed desires and the somatic translation of those desires into bodily misbehaviours – yet the history of hysteria suggests broader transmogrifications as well. What if hysterical behaviour has indeed been for some a sort of coded language, a language of desires made unattainable by the social conditions into which those desires were born? What if, historically, women had no words for their frustrations and their desires because no such words were allowed, and because their subordination was such that such words were not to be heard? This would begin to explain the misattribution of hysteria to wombs and witches; it would also confirm that the real issue was the mistranslation of women's emotional and bodily language – the misunderstanding of their 'hysterical' medium of communication – by male interpreters. More broadly, it would suggest that whatever its individual manifestations, the distortions of hysteria emerge in the fraught interplay of social structure, social relationships, and situated biography.

This is precisely the approach that Schuilenburg employs, and it forms the thematic core of his book. Hysteria, he writes, is 'above all a sociological issue', and because of this, the aim of the book is 'to bring to light previously hidden relationships in our society. As a result, reality is reordered in a way that leads to the emergence of new connections, and to a redefinition of hysteria and the way it affects our society today more than ever.' For Schuilenburg, this sociology of hysteria becomes a sort of sociological mystery story, as he searches for these hidden relationships and emerging connections – and one of the real strengths of the book is the breadth and depth of his search. He conducts an ethnographic inquiry into a contemporary immigrant neighbourhood in Rotterdam, and excavates a Rotterdam race riot from the 1970s – but he also explores other places and other times in a way that makes the book soundly international and comparative. He thoughtfully revisits and reconsiders philosophical traditions from Hobbes to Hume to De Waal – but he also finds clues in the less august worlds of popular music, film, and science fiction. Time and again, he shows that to situate hysteria in social relations, we must consider long-standing traditions, contemporary popular culture, and emerging global dynamics. In doing so, he persuasively makes the case that, while hysteria may have been erased from psychiatry's *Diagnostic and Statistical Manual* and discarded as a legitimate medical diagnosis, it continues to circulate wildly in the world at large.

Hysteria also moves beyond individual pathology and into the realm of the social to the extent that it is performative. As Schuilenburg notes, hysteria can in many cases be understood as a 'scream for recognition' or a 'cry for meaning', a desperate demand that the pain and frustration of existence be acknowledged. In this sense hysteria is performed, with the hope that this performance will find a sympathetic audience. Here we see a fascinating example of the contemporary 'will-to-representation', in Majid Yar's (2012) term – the deep yearning to be seen and acknowledged – and with this a 'dramaturgy of social life' (Goffman 1956) that implicates actor and audience alike. Understood in this way, hysteria fits all too comfortably with a contemporary world of cell phone selfies, personal YouTube channels, TikTok videos, and digital confessionals; its frantic staging defines it as less an aberration than yet another performance amidst a social life shaped by performance. Of course, like other performances, a hysterical performance may generate an empathic audience attuned to its cry for meaning, or it may produce an audience that judges it to be outlandish, overwrought, even threatening. In the theatre of the absurd that is hysteria, and that is contemporary social life, actor and audience form yet another fraught relationship.

The prevalence of hysterical performance in contemporary social life begins to reveal still other hidden relationships of the sort that Schuilenburg seeks to explain. Late modernity offers us an existence in which the certainty of stable work life and career, the security of a foundational belief system, and the clarity of truth versus falsehood have all but disappeared. As Jock Young (2007, p. 13) argues, some find in this anomic disorder the seeds of liberation and renewal, others the justification for punitive exclusion and fundamentalism – but almost all find in it a disconcerting dizziness, a 'late modern vertigo' brought on by 'insecurities of status and of economic position'. This vertigo, and with it a fear of falling through the cracks in the social order, in turn produce excesses of expressive emotion, desperate searches for self-identity, and hysterical displays of discomfort and despair. In this late modern world more and more people find themselves cast adrift not only from normative certainty but from geographic stability as well, living their lives as perpetual and unwelcome outsiders, and forced to invent what fragile forms of community they can. 'Intensities of ephemeral association' (Ferrell 2018, p. 18) result, with status negotiated in the moment, relationships found and lost, and emotions exacerbated by the brevity of their duration. In comparison to those privileged to retain a more sedentary existence, the lives of those adrift are animated by the heightened excitement of the moment and the frisson of ongoing uncertainty. From the perspective of the sedentary, the lived experiences of those adrift no doubt seem hysterical – and in many ways, they are. A social system of vertiginous doubt leaves many of its citizens little but hysteria in response.

In confronting this swirling late modern world and its hysterical currents, we might well wish to take measures that would introduce a modicum of calm and security; we might even hope to knit back the social fabric so as to restore a sense of Durkheimian social cohesion. But it is here that Schuilenburg drops an anomic bomb, delivering with it one of his most important insights: In the contemporary world, attempts to confront and calm hysteria generally have the effect of exacerbating it. Schuilenburg's Rotterdam neighbourhood ethnography, for example, focuses on a governmental Neighbourhood Takes Charge (NTC) initiative designed to strengthen neighbourhood solidarity and promote participation in local governance. As the programme progresses, though, neighbourhood frustration only increases, with building anger at the city government's lack of response to local NTC recommendations and ever more hysterical NTC meetings. More broadly, contemporary 'wars on crime' and 'wars on drugs' constitute hysterical, alarmist publicity campaigns rather than careful policy programmes; not surprisingly, they in turn promote panic over crime and fantastic, fearful caricatures of criminals and drug users. All of this, Schuilenburg argues, creates a sort of 'security hysteria' where security policies based on manufactured fear and political expediency create a downward spiral whereby 'phantom security' spawns only greater fear and hysteria. In this dynamic we see yet again 'the ironies of social control' (Marx 1981), and yet again the process that labelling theorists have long understood, whereby 'social control leads to deviance' (Lemert 1967: v). Assuming we wish to occupy a relatively non-hysterical world, this endless amplification of hysteria would be sufficient cause for concern – but then Schuilenburg exposes a further irony: The 'success paradox', whereby 'the wealthier, healthier and safer our lives become, the more hysterical the last residue of lack makes us feel'.

Hysteria, it seems, is a permanent and pervasive social phenomenon, at least for those occupying what's left of the first world. Still other features of that world only reinforce late modernity's rampant hysteria. Digital media not only promote mediated performance; they also promote self-reinforcing intensities of shared emotion, and they profit from algorithmically-enhanced irrationality. In this sense social media function to spread the infection of hysteria, creating an ongoing collectivity of misinformation and emotional volatility. More traditional forms of media do their part as well, promoting the over-the-top drama of 'reality' television shows, constructing news programming around the sorts of sensationalist stories that will maximise ratings and profit, and fostering a culture in which transgression and punishment are consumed for their illicit titillations (Binik 2020; Brown 2009). Consumer culture itself operates on the endless manufacture of need and desire, with the false promise of fulfilment by this product and the next, until the consumer's material insatiability grows into an insatiability of being. Politically, the recent emergence of right-wing populism runs on organised resentment, and with it a penchant for aggressive irrationality and overblown violence – the result being a deathly cult of authoritarian personality that denies not only science but the very possibility of inclusive sociality.

So, with a certain tremble in our voice, we might well ask: What is to become of us? Two trajectories would seem plausible, both grounded in social dynamics. In the first, hysteria accelerates to the point that it emerges as the new template for normality. Perhaps hysteria has in fact already become the lingua franca of the late modern world, the common and expected medium for politics, entertainment, and communication. After all, emotions can only be judged over-the-top, behaviours only condemned as excessively attention-seeking, political arguments only dismissed as irrational in comparison to some baseline of calm consideration. But if that baseline has been obliterated by pervasive contemporary hysteria, can the alleged deviance of individual hysteria still exist? In conditions of pervasive bedlam, after all, the chaos can hardly be traced to any one voice. Or, to paraphrase Durkheim, while a saintly society may still harbour deviance, it's not at all clear that a hysterical society will continue to harbour hysterics.

But there's a second tantalising possibility, one with which Schuilenburg ends the book: the possibility that hysteria might hold a bit of revolutionary spark, and with it a portent of change in the contemporary social order. If hysteria can operate as a coded language of repressed desire, perhaps it can also operate as an inchoate language of social distress; perhaps those we deem hysterics are those left to twist, shout, and sputter against a social system made increasingly unbearable. As that system continues to spin out of control, widespread hysteria would suggest that the horrors of that system transcend the ability to speak fully of them – and that a coherent language of a new world is yet to be coined. To paraphrase Gramsci, as the old world dies and the new world waits to emerge, hysteria may be one of the 'morbid symptoms' that flourishes in the interregnum. If so, hysteria may hold a tellingly interstitial position, emerging from the contemporary crisis but not fully conversant with it, and like Simmel's (1971) 'stranger', part of the present world but anticipating alternatives to it. If this is the case, then as Schuilenburg says, perhaps 'certain issues should be treated with a little less hysteria, while others could do with some more'.

Note

1 At around this same time Cesare Lombroso was likewise performatively exhibiting the new "science" of criminology in Italy; see Morrison (2004).

References

Binik, O. (2020). *The Fascination with Violence in Contemporary Society*. Cham, Switzerland: Palgrave Macmillan.

Brown, M. (2009). *The Culture of Punishment*. New York: New York University Press.

Ferrell, J. (2018). *Drift: Illicit Mobility and Uncertain Knowledge*. Oakland, CA: University of California Press.

Goffman, E. (1956). *The Presentation of Self in Everyday Life*. New York: Doubleday.

Lemert, E. (1967). *Human Deviance, Social Problems and Social Control*. Englewood Cliffs, NJ: Prentice Hall.

Marx, G. (1981). Ironies of Social Control: Authorities as Contributors to Deviance through Escalation, Nonenforcement and Covert Facilitation. *Social Problems*, 28(3): 221–246.

Morrison, W. (2004). Lombroso and the Birth of Criminological Positivism. In J. Ferrell *et al.* (eds), *Cultural Criminology Unleashed* (pp. 67–80). London: Glasshouse.

Simmel, G. (1971 [1908]). The Stranger. In D. Levine (ed.), *Georg Simmel: On Individuality and Social Forms* (pp. 143–149). Chicago, IL: University of Chicago Press.

Yar, M. (2012). Crime, Media and the Will-to-Representation: Reconsidering Relationships in the New Media Age. *Crime, Media, Culture*, 8(3): 245–260.

Young, J. (2007). *The Vertigo of Late Modernity*. London: Sage.

Here, the facts are hysterical.

David Wallace-Wells, *The Uninhabitable Earth: Life After Warming*

The hysteric is at the same time someone who imposes his or her presence, but also someone for whom things and beings are present, too present, and who attributes to everything and communicates to every being this excessive presence.

Gilles Deleuze, *Francis Bacon: The Logic of Sensation*

Chapter 1

Hysteria is dead, long live hysteria

Hysteria has gone the way of the dodo. Vanished from our society, the illness has been consigned to the landfill of Western history. It happened in the 1980s, when hysteria was deleted from the *Diagnostic and Statistical Manual of Mental Disorders* (DSM), the diagnostic and statistical manual of psychiatric disorders used by psychologists and doctors worldwide to diagnose psychiatric conditions. The entry 'hysterical personality', for example, has been replaced by 'histrionic personality'. In editions following the third (DSM-III, from 1980), hysteria appears only residually within smaller groups of everyday conditions such as psychosis, personality disorders, conversion and dissociation. It is difficult to determine with hindsight why hysteria was removed from the DSM, though it seems that there was no consensus in the medical world on how to define the condition. Should it be described as pain in certain parts of the body for which no clear cause can be found, or as an aetiological process, linked with the patient's subconscious? What we do know, is that the disappearance of hysteria has something to do with the – originally American – DSM's anti-psychoanalytical stance, and the strongly diminished popularity of Sigmund Freud's work, which revolved to an important degree around hysteria. This is reflected by the fact that Freud's work is no longer required reading at universities, and his theories are hardly ever applied in practice anymore. Many no longer even consider Freud a scientist, but see in him an exposed charlatan and fantasist.[1] A persistent rumour has it that the editors of the DSM at the University of Washington even put up a photograph of the maligned Freud above the urinals in the men's room. The only places Freud's psychoanalysis is still alive and kicking are popular culture and the literary world.

We also know that hysteria's fall from grace in the medical world coincided with the rise of evidence-based thinking. This school of thought, which emerged in the early 1980s, has strong reservations about psychoanalysis's non-testable axioms and the dubious validity of its diagnostic methods. Instead, it leans strongly towards applications with well-defined and limited objectives whose efficacy have been unequivocally proven. Scientific proof has replaced the expertise of physicians, based on the premise that if something cannot be measured, it does not exist. In addition, psychoanalysis was surpassed in popularity by cognitive behavioural therapy in the 1980s, a method that concentrates not on where negative feelings like anger and frustration come from, but on how to deal with them. It is based on the idea that every situation is processed cognitively, and that this process determines our behaviour and emotions. This means that the way you perceive things has an important influence on your behavioural patterns. Learning to control your emotions and to interpret events differently gives you a more objective view of your own perceptions, which allows you to eliminate unpleasant feelings and change your behaviour for the better.

In line with the celebrated evidenced-based thinking, and in stark contrast with the negative image of psychoanalysis, cognitive behavioural therapy was thought to be firmly scientifically grounded in empirically verified procedures. What's more, cognitive behavioural therapy had the important advantage of being substantially cheaper and more efficient than psychoanalysis. While psychoanalysis relies on providing a patient with time and space to say everything that is on their mind during a lengthy course of therapy, cognitive behavioural therapy is a short-term treatment, consisting of between 10 and 20 sessions on average. By comparison, psychoanalysis requires weekly sessions on the therapist's couch, exploring the deeper layers of the patient's subconscious, for a period of between three and five years. The time and cost involved in this treatment make it the preserve of the upper classes, as an average course of psychoanalysis costs €12,500 annually – and that for a minimum of three years.

All this gives the impression that hysteria became extinct at the end of the 20th century. In his book *Histoire de l'hystérie* from 1986, the French medical historian Étienne Trillat writes that 'there can be no doubt that hysteria is dead [...], and that it has taken its secrets to the grave with it'.[2] At least, so it seems – but looks can be deceiving. You only have to turn on the television or go online to recognise Western culture's most basic ingredient: hysteria is everywhere. Whether in the worldwide run on toilet paper amid the coronavirus crisis, the discussion about Black Pete reaching its annual fever pitch in the Netherlands, the madness of the wildly fluctuating housing market, or the heated debates about climate change, hysteria dominates the world stage. It pops up so frequently that hardly a day goes by on which it does not make an appearance. Be it in the papers, on television, in everyday conversations or in politics, the image of citizens and politicians displaying over-the-top emotional reactions is sure to grab the public's attention. The striking thing about this is that hysteria is not limited to a small group of people, on the contrary; large groups in particular seem increasingly to fall prey to it. We become hysterical because so many others are hysterical. This is not so much the result of time and place, but of a collective contamination through social networks – an observation that goes back to the work of the 19th-century French sociologist Gabriel Tarde on how the invention of the printing press and the telegraph brought people closer together.[3] Facebook and Twitter, platforms on which hysteria spreads like an infectious disease, clearly show how this collective contagion works. It is even arguable that hysteria is an inherent part of Twitter. In the often overheated discussions on the platform, Twitter hooligans foist themselves on each other, bandying about tweets full of the necessary capital letters, exclamation marks and moving GIFs, supplemented with the famous crying smileys and laughing turds.

Hysteria may have been scrapped from the DSM, but it is more widespread than ever in daily life. The frenzied tenor of our society becomes especially noticeable in our handling of such subjects as security, health, identity, immigration and wealth. Despite their apparent differences, these subjects have in common that they all display hysterical traits. Not because they are hysterical in themselves, but in the sense that they are in some strange way permeated with hysterical characteristics. At the risk of generalising, security policies can be seen as an example of our habitually overwrought reaction to the levels of crime and disorder around us. Despite living in the safest society in history, many people believe it is less safe than ever before. Opening a random newspaper, you will find the daily headlines are dominated by crime and disorder, creating an atmosphere of constant panic. Alternately, ask any minister for their opinion on their country's safety, and they will tell you all about how unsafe it is and that unless heavier sentences and more stringent measures are implemented, criminals will be given 'free rein'. Western countries are thought to be plagued by crime, with robberies and burglaries being the order of the day. As a result of this, we have been flooded by a veritable tsunami of new laws and measures to fight crime and disorder in recent years. This liquid policy – to paraphrase Zygmunt Bauman – is in fact nothing short of a Sisyphean task. Not a week goes by without the Ministry of Justice coming up with yet another measure to tackle the country's security issues; it is hard to keep track.

All of this stands in stark contrast to the fact that crime rates in Western countries have fallen spectacularly for years. In the Netherlands, for instance, registered and victim-reported crime has dropped by about 30% since 2002, and the number of registered offences is at its lowest point in almost forty years. This applies to almost all types of offences, ranging from car theft to burglary and from robberies to vandalism, while the number of homicides has more than halved in the past decade. This is not only true for the Netherlands, the same pattern can be discerned in other European countries and the United States. In other words, the punitive populism that is pushing ever more stringent security policies is completely out of kilter with the actual improvements in safety and security. This raises the question why more and more money is spent on surveillance measures based on the presumption that people cannot be trusted, such as CCTV cameras and zero tolerance, which are not only expensive but actually very ineffective. There is no debate about this.

To put the same problem another way: objectively speaking, life has never been better, but that is not how we perceive it. In a country that has never been wealthier, many people worry excessively about the future. This is remarkable, given that Western countries are among the richest in the world. Nor is it a recent development – Norway, Luxembourg, Ireland and the Netherlands have been close to the top of the world's wealthiest countries for a long time, and not only in terms of hard finances and narrow prosperity; as the economy expands and people's spending power increases, prosperity grows wider. Almost all social indicators such as our life expectancy, level of education, employment rate, and trust in other people are positive, but the average citizen's gut feeling ignores these reassuring statistics. Put bluntly, people simply don't buy it. They do not believe things are getting any better at all, and view good news with suspicion. Statistics are just figures, and hysteria has no respect whatsoever for facts. Fake news, or, as David Byrne puts it in the song 'Crosseyed and Painless': 'Facts just twist the truth around.' Citizens distrust government statistics, which they believe show biased results. An often-heard mantra is 'They can't fool me.' A large part of the population have serious concerns about society going downhill, talking about the hooliganisation of society and the decline of community spirit. They project their worries onto groups and institutions coming from 'abroad' that don't 'belong' into our habitat: immigrants, Muslims and the European Union have all come under fire.

In many respects, humanity is doing better all the time, yet this is not our perception. There is a gaping chasm between the figures and statistics on the population's happiness and well-being on the one hand, and the alarmist tone in which the Apocalypse is announced on the other. This raises the question how today's hysteria should be understood. In daily life, the term hysteria generally has negative connotations. It refers to a state of mind of someone who has lost their senses, is displaying extreme behaviour and refuses to see reason. You could also say that hysteria and reason do not go well together. The term has pejorative connotations and is usually used to refer to a person's overwrought personality. This theatrical trait of hysteria is the first thing most people will answer if asked to describe a hysterical person. A hysteric is someone with high spirits, frequent mood swings and a very quick temper – the kind of people who are always told not to 'be hysterical'. Women often bear the brunt of this, being far more likely than men to be accused of hysteria: while a silent man is considered deep, an outspoken woman is hysterical. The history of the disease teaches that young or unstable women, widows and women with an overly strong and insufficiently satisfied sex drive are thought to be especially prone to hysteria.

Like no other philosopher before him, Michel Foucault has shown that Western history has its own unique diseases. In *History of Madness*, published in 1961 as *Folie et déraison*, he distinguishes between three historical periods, each marked by its own inner logic and standards of truth-seeking: the Renaissance, the Classical age, and modernity. In *Histoire de la folie à l'âge classique*, Foucault describes how madness was perceived in the Renaissance and in the 17th and 18th centuries, which he calls *l'âge classique*, interpreting this perception as the effect of a discourse which gives coherence and meaning to the way of thinking and acting in such a historical period. The French word *folie* can mean 'madness' as well as 'foolishness'. In the Renaissance, when the two meanings were closely related, madness was considered simply a part of life, an inherent part of society, which was connected to the metaphysical, magical world. The tragic aspect of madness was based on its ever-presence in the guise of countless frightening and fascinating creatures, as Hieronymus Bosch depicted magnificently in his apocalyptic drawings and paintings, culminating in *The Garden of Earthly Delights* from 1480–1490. Another representation of *folie* can be found in *Dulle Griet* by Peter Bruegel the Elder, in which it is depicted as madness. The Rijksmuseum in Amsterdam and the National Gallery in London are full of mid-17th-century engravings that show people suffering from some form of madness.

In the Classical age, the period following the Renaissance, a completely different view on madness gained ground. Madness evolved from something intangible into a *maladie mentale*, a medical syndrome. Foucault calls this an analytical or more critical approach, in which madness is viewed as a purely medical phenomenon that refers to nothing but itself. One important explanation for the emergence of this analytical approach is that it was the first time in history that humans formulated a rational discourse of themselves as a subject of knowledge. People came to view themselves as rational, calculating citizens. An example of this is Descartes' insight that as long as we think rationally, we cannot be insane, which prompted Foucault to write that the Cartesian step towards doubt is an attempt to ward off insanity. Madness turned into the denial of reason and assumed the value of irrationality. You could also say that madness and reason were no longer engaging in a meaningful dialogue. Isolated and kept at a safe distance, it was placed outside of the prevailing morals of the day, where it no longer posed a threat to reason. Madness was silenced by what Foucault called 'the big lock-up', in which anyone who was strange or different was locked away in workhouses, hospitals, detention centres, prisons, mental institutions and halfway houses – the so-called *hôpitaux généraux*. In this way, both crime and madness were banished from society by treating them behind closed doors.

In a development closely associated with the banishment of madness, a medical outlook emerged which differentiated between various forms of insanity, including melancholy, hypochondria and hysteria. This new perspective, in which hysteria was entered in a moral-medical model and increasingly referred to in medical terms, was characterised by a rejection of classificatory knowledge. The relationships within this classic form of knowledge are structured like the family tree of a large family: a symptom is assigned to an illness, an illness to a species group and a species group to the greater pathological framework. Each classification comes with its specific treatment that gave the physician precise instructions on what to do. This universal method of treatment was thought to solve all of the patients' problems. In *The Birth of the Clinic*, Foucault writes about a hysterical woman being treated for ten months with daily baths that lasted between ten and twelve hours. In the course of the 18th century, classificatory rule, which dominated medical theory and practice, was gradually replaced by the more positive, empirical knowledge of anatomical medicine. During this revolution in medical thinking, which according to Foucault took place between 1780 and 1820, hysteria broke away from the metaphysics of evil as well as from Satan and the demons with which it had been associated until that time.

This new medical approach made structural deviations in individual cases of hysteria possible for the first time. Naturally, patients suffering from the condition still showed countless similarities, but the essence of the illness now lay in its localisability, in the possibility of pinpointing its exact location in the body. But while the seat of the illness could now be determined in every patient individually, this required looking at the bigger picture: the patient's own history, his or her personality, information about their life, environment, family, and much more. This was part of a wider trend in medical thinking, which no longer aimed to fit all conditions into one table in an unambiguous system listing the conditions' characteristics as well as possible interventions. Physicians now saw their patients, in the literal sense, as people with individual pathological histories which needed to be unravelled before their hysteria could be treated effectively. The closed structures of classificatory knowledge were replaced by series of boundless, endless tables. Foucault writes:

> What now constituted the unity of the medical gaze was not the circle of knowledge in which it was achieved but that open, infinite, moving totality, ceaselessly displaced and enriched by time, whose course it began but would never be able to stop.[4]

The reversal of the medical discourse was rounded off by the way in which patients were allowed to express themselves in the psychiatrist's office of Sigmund Freud. Using free association, the technique that succeeded hypnosis, Freud encouraged his patients to speak freely and spontaneously about anything that came into their heads, and to indicate which of their past experiences had had an emotional impact, however hard they may have found it.

While Freud, a self-declared admirer of author and physician Sir Arthur Conan Doyle and his *Adventures of Sherlock Holmes*, searched for his patients' deepest secrets like a private detective so as to let them relive their repressed memories, I will consider the problem of hysteria from a different angle. Instead of searching for the secret of hysteria, I want to find out why it continues to operate in our society. General practitioners are increasingly raising the alarm about the growing number of patients with complaints that are very similar to hysteria symptoms, often in combination with depression, ADHD, burnout and stress. All of these illnesses have of course always existed, but the number of adults who suffer from them has risen since the turn of the century. In fact, besides being one of the happiest countries on earth, the Netherlands is also in the top 10 of countries with the highest number of inhabitants suffering from depression. As many as one in five Dutch adults is affected by depressive episodes every year, in many cases as a result of stress, and takes antidepressants. That makes roughly 550,000 Dutch people who suffer from unhappiness, while according to the World Health Organisation, depression affects over 300 million people worldwide.

Hysterical people can be irritating or fascinating, but leave hardly anyone indifferent. Despite our deep fascination with all aspects of hysteria, however, it is not so well known as not to need an introduction. In fact, its meaning is still unclear and controversial today. Hysteria has been an exceptionally vague concept throughout history, which has caused plenty of confusion, and even doubt about whether it has ever existed. The Belgian psychologist Paul Verhaeghe writes that 'no other phenomenon has triggered such a wide-ranging variety of theories'.[5] Medical and historical researchers, psychoanalyst and philosophers, religious and gender studies as well as painters, writers and film producers have all engaged with hysteria and tried to unravel its mysteries. From a historical perspective, we know hysteria from stories about cursed women possessed by the devil who were burnt at the stake as witches. From ancient Egyptian times until deep into the 18th century, hysteria was diagnosed as a convulsive disorder, and the womb cast as the villain of the piece. The thinking behind this was that hysteria was caused by the womb, which was believed to move freely throughout the body all the way into the head, emitting toxic fumes that led to hysteria. The condition has also been examined through a psychoanalytic lens, Freud's work being the most famous example. While many of his ideas have become irrelevant, such as his fixation on the Oedipus complex which is no longer taken seriously today, a theory of his that still resonates with us is that hysteria is caused by traumatic events that cannot be put into words and are expressed instead through bodily complaints. Feminist thinkers such as Hélène Cixous, Catherine Clément and Luce Irigaray, for example, have regarded hysteria as a female system of meaning outside official languages and cultural conventions. They consider hysterical symptoms to be a rebellion against the social and institutional order of our society, which restricts women especially in their freedom. 'What woman is not Dora?', Cixous asks in *The Newly-Born Woman* from 1986, referring to Freud's famous case history of the 18-year-old Dora, a persistent hysteria sufferer.

That is not to say, however, that it is absolutely necessary to read Freud's work to study hysteria. Hysterics come in all shapes and sizes. You get them in politics and in the sciences, and the arts and literature are also swarming with hysterical people. You find hysteria in the dysmorphic screaming figures of the Irish painter Francis Bacon, such as his portrait of Pope Innocent X. Gilles Deleuze describes the paintings as hysterical for the numerous characteristics of hysteria they depict, such as violent muscle spasms and cramps, and even claims there is a special relationship between hysteria and painting. In his 1981 study *Francis Bacon*, he writes about the 'hysterical essence of painting', by which he means the presence of sensations in painting that cannot be reduced to a representation, as this would automatically sideline them.[6] It almost goes without saying that hysteria exerts an irresistible pull on literature as well. In his novella *Fanny* from 1879, the Dutch author Marcellus Emants portrays his wife as an extremely irritable and nervous woman suffering from frequent mood swings, while other literary examples featuring hysteria include Flaubert's *Madame Bovary* (1856), Tolstoy's *Anna Karenina* (1877) and Couperus's *Eline Vere* (1889). Hysteria has leading roles in Hollywood, too. We love movies that feature hysteria or characters with hysterical disorders, such as *A Dangerous Method* (2011), which examines the relationship between the psychiatrist Carl Jung and his mentally ill patient Sabina Spielrein. 'Do I really look like a guy with a plan?' cries the perpetually grinning Joker, played by Heath Ledger, in *The Dark Knight* (2008) by Christopher Nolan. His unique talent for disrupting the status quo ('You know, I just … do things') and his favourite weapon of a poison from which people die while laughing hysterically and are left with a Joker-like grin on their faces give the Joker an enduring appeal to our imaginations. In her eponymous book, Elaine Showalter calls these cultural narratives of hysteria 'hystories'.[7]

Plenty of reasons, it seems, to focus our attention on hysteria. So why has hysteria as a medical diagnosis been removed from the DSM? Does hysteria only affect women, or can men be hysterical too? What is the role of hysteria in such issues as security and immigration? How can people fall into such a delirium? What does hysteria tell us about our way of life? In short, what can hysteria mean to modern thought? In this book, I will try to answer the above questions and more. The answers can be found by searching for the psychological factors connected to hysteria. This is the classical approach, which considers hysteria a purely 'stand-alone' phenomenon that can be clinically and diagnostically analysed. A more modern approach focuses on biological factors such as genetic variations which make some people more prone to hysteria than others. While not wishing to detract from either approach, I have no intention of examining them in detail, as that would only heighten the mystery of hysteria; so many studies have already been published on both sides of the story that it would be impossible to do them justice. Besides, the psychological and biological factors displayed are different for every hysteric, and both factors can change in the course of a life. But even more importantly, I believe that a different approach can explain more about hysteria than explanations focused on a single factor or a combination of psychological and biological factors. For hysteria is also and above all a sociological issue. The problem of hysteria is sociologically relevant because it raises the question of why our lives, which seem to run so smoothly for many people, are nevertheless so hysterical.

I will therefore attempt to make a sociological analysis of hysteria in order to understand why this illness crops up so often and in such diverging fields, ranging from the issue of safety and security to the arrival of immigrants and asylum seekers. I will base my analysis on the broader meaning of the word 'hysteria', which emphasises the extraordinarily overwrought tone in which people express themselves on the one hand, and the conflicts about political and moral issues that gave rise to it, such as security and immigration, on the other. In this view, hysteria serves as an organising concept that can help us understand our world and ourselves. In his main work *Difference and Repetition*, Deleuze describes this method as a combination of 'a very particular species of detective novel, in part a kind of science fiction'.[8] A private detective works in a strictly empirical fashion, by searching for clues to fathom the mysteries of hysteria. Just like a philosopher, the detective makes all kinds of connections during his search, trying to piece together an understanding of the illness before all the details have become clear. He consults experts in his quest to shed light on the disappearance of hysteria from the DSM, peruses witness reports on widespread outbreaks of hysteria in the media, subjects the medical murder weapon with which hysteria was killed to fresh scrutiny, and finally conducts an extensive crime scene investigation to find out whether the conflicts that cause hysteria have really disappeared. It is important to note that this method does not focus exclusively on reconstructing the past, in the way that Sherlock Holmes uncovers the absolute truth by scientifically tracking down and piecing together missing clues in Sir Arthur Conan Doyle's classic detective stories. The aim is, rather, to bring to light previously hidden relationships in our society. As a result, reality is reordered in a way that leads to the emergence of new connections, and to a redefinition of hysteria and the way it affects our society today more than ever.

This perspective, which allows us to view society and ourselves in a different light, is also the link with the science fiction genre. William Gibson, the author of the 1984 novel *Neuromancer*, which inspired the Matrix trilogy directed by Lana and Lilly Wachowski, describes science fiction as a way of pre-programming the present. Despite appearing to be ahead of the times, the genre primarily deals with the present, projecting issues that occupy us now onto the near future. This opens a window on another world, as it were, allowing us a much closer look at today's world and preparing us for times that are still to come. Thinking from a future perspective, we are able to shape our own future instead of constantly trying to keep up, which highlights just how relevant the future is to the present.[9] If we want to understand what hysteria is, we need to recognise that it constitutes an inherent part of our culture – not the sudden movements and speech impediments, the typical paralysis, nervous coughs and ticks of the hysterical person, but an analysis of wider developments in our society which enable hysteria to continue to function, and to do so in ever-changing fields and ever-changing guises. After all, if hysteria is an informative part of our society, society itself needs to be examined: why is it appearing at this moment, after these events, in this period?

A 'whodunit', in other words, laced with science fiction disguised as sociology. Not wanting to limit myself to an abstract quest for hysteria, however, I have tried also to delve deeper into the subject through other methods, and would like to conclude this introduction with a brief summary of them. One thing I have always found dissatisfying in the works of such philosophers as Michel Foucault and Gilles Deleuze is that they contain hardly any people of flesh and blood. In his books on madness and the modern prison, Foucault refers to people, their emotions and feelings exclusively in abstract terms like 'the insane', 'psychiatric experts' and 'delinquents'. As a result, his analysis no longer bears any relation to the very people Foucault claims to be making a stand for: the detained and the insane. His interest in madness, for example, focuses mainly on its meaning as represented in texts on insanity of a certain period, such as medical writings or the works of philosophers, poets, writers and painters from the 17th and 18th centuries. As a result of this archaeological method, insanity becomes completely detached from the insane themselves, the people who actually live with hysteria and experience it on a daily basis. Foucault makes an artificial distinction between the living environment of the insane on the one hand and the way in which these people are represented in texts and writings on the other. This distinction does not do justice to the fact that in reality, the two worlds cannot be separated from one another − each world determines the form, content and meaning of the other. What is more, the lives of the 'insane' do not come to life merely from descriptions categorised under such lifeless terms as 'mentally ill' and 'imbecilic'. This means that while Foucault's analysis of hysteria may be correct from an ideal-typical perspective, it can be wide of the mark empirically.

For this reason, I have decided not to approach hysteria as an abstract social phenomenon, but to examine what makes the condition pop up in different locations time and again, and why people are gripped so quickly by the sudden excitement and excessive emotions it causes. A practice-based sociological research like this one does not start at the library, but on the street. One of the methods I have used is ethnographic research. Reasoning from hysteria also means experiencing first hand why emotions run so high among citizens when it comes to government policies and interventions in such concrete situations as improving the liveability of big cities, which is why I have spent two years doing research in the socially deprived Rotterdam neighbourhood Hillesluis, to observe up close where the residents' agitation comes from. In Hillesluis, I was a member of *Buurt Bestuurt* (Neighbourhood Takes Charge), a new initiative which gives residents a say in the development of council and police policies, and involves them in their implementation. It is based on the presumption that no one is better qualified to know what a neighbourhood needs to become 'clean, intact and safe' than its residents. During my two years as a member of this initiative, I interviewed the participants in the hope of gaining a better understanding of their anger and main frustrations about the liveability in their neighbourhood. But I also spoke with people on the street, I sat on benches in public squares, held surveys and visited social activities in Hillesluis in an effort to penetrate to the heart of this Rotterdam problem neighbourhood. This has allowed me to experience first-hand why the residents think that the liveability in their neighbourhood is so bad and why they believe the actions of council and police are seriously flawed and failing in their duty to the public.

In addition to chapters devoted to themes like liveability and security, I will also discuss the arrival of asylum seekers and immigrants, and examine the language of hysteria. Two subjects that stir up public opinion like no others, immigration and security, are often mentioned in the same breath, as if immigration implied a threat to security. August 1972 marked a significant date in the debate on immigration in the Netherlands, when the country's first race riots took place in the South Rotterdam Afrikaander neighbourhood. As a result of the riots, Rotterdam was one of the first Dutch municipalities to address the question of how we should handle the arrival of foreigners to our country. This presents a perfect opportunity for reflection, and for comparing the debate on the race riots with today's overwrought discussion on the admission and naturalisation of newcomers to Western countries. For the language used in such debates is anything but an innocent phenomenon. Apart from being a beautiful and powerful medium for describing reality, language is also a tool for shaping that reality, in that it can determine the view we take of a subject and lead our actions. While the immortal words of the French poet and critic Stéphane Mallarmé, 'to change language is to change the world', may be a slight exaggeration, they do contain a kernel of truth.

This book is organised as follows. Chapter 2 is a largely descriptive account of the thinking on the causes of hysteria throughout the ages by physicians, psychologists, philosophers and other scientists, ranging from Plato to Freud and everything in between. I have not attempted to give a comprehensive view of all philosophical, psychological and medical theories that exist on this subject. Instead, I will discuss a number of interpretations in the history of hysteria that have been at the forefront of our thinking about this disease, including a somatic, a paranormal and a psychological explanation. In Chapter 3, I will focus on hysterical attitudes to security, and show that it is closely linked to our inherent tendency to think of security in terms of war. If security is a story, it is one told in the language of warfare: 'war on drugs', 'war on terror', 'war on crime', 'war on corona'. In an analysis of Thomas Hobbes's work, I will show how his notion of a constant 'war of all against all' laid the foundation for our hysterical attitude towards the last remnants of danger left in our society today.

In my criticism of Hobbes's negative, almost animalistic view of humanity, I will subsequently discuss the scientific debate on such positive emotions as empathy and altruism. The internationally known Dutch primatologist and ethologist Frans De Waal, one of the fiercest critics of Hobbes's school of thought and its followers, rejects that humans are animalistic savages who are constantly out to bash each other's brains in, arguing that such capacities as empathy and altruism are over one hundred million years old and deeply anchored in human nature. In Chapter 4, I will substantiate that De Waal's work points the way to a different, less hysterical image of the relationship between safety and life. I call this positive security.

In Chapter 5, on the communications revolution of social media, I argue that our relationship with social media borders on the hysterical. Many people seem to have completely lost control of the amount of time they spend on them. We check our phones first thing in the morning and take it to bed at night. A quick look on Twitter, a quick post on Instagram, check Facebook to see what is going on: we constantly feel under pressure not to miss anything and to respond to each and every message. But seeing is being seen – messages and conversations on Facebook and Twitter also provide useful information for tracking down potential criminals. Our hysterical online life allows investigation authorities to predict crimes. My quest to understand how hysteria works continues in Chapter 6, an empirical chapter about the two years I spent as a member of Neighbourhood Takes Charge, in which Hillesluis residents give an extensive account of the actual influence that Neighbourhood Takes Charge gives them on the approach to tackling the neighbourhood's greatest problems. They talk about the city council's reluctance to cooperate and the red tape they encountered on every step of the way, and in the picture that emerges from the interviews, frustration and anger heap up and lead to a deeply entrenched resentment against the government.

Chapter 7 discusses hysterical hyperboles in the debate about immigration. To give language its proper place in the thinking about hysteria, I delved into the archives of the Rotterdam city council to sift through the discussions that took place in the press and politics after fighting had broken out between Dutch and Turkish residents of the Afrikaander neighbourhood. In August 1972, the Rotterdam Afrikaander neighbourhood made international headlines when riots erupted that lasted almost a week. A conflict over unpaid rent between a Turkish landlord and his Dutch tenant got completely out of hand and descended into a sudden and unprecedented explosion of public anger against the neighbourhood's Turkish inhabitants and the local police. The race riots, as the newspapers and television called them, and the political discussion they sparked in the city council, shed an interesting light on the current discussion about immigration and integration and the subject of moral panic. Finally, the book concludes in Chapter 8 with a reflection on the most important insight that my quest in the preceding chapters has yielded, showing that hysteria has become a business model. While, medically speaking, hysteria no longer exists, politics, the economy and social media still profit from the occasional panic. I introduce the success paradox and show the difference between destructive and constructive hysteria, and how the latter rouses people to take action and can lead to wide-reaching social changes. In this way, hysteria can be both terrible and useful.

The DSM, the bible of psychiatry, advises not to fear hysteria, since it does not exist. But while psychologists and physicians claim that hysteria is a thing of the past, an outdated diagnosis that has disappeared for good, this book argues that it is in fact alive and well. Hyperventilating, we rush from one incident into the next – there is hardly time for a breather. The debate on crime or immigration comes to a head at the slightest provocation. Irritating though this may be, hysteria needs to be taken seriously, for what it tells us about our society and way of life.

Notes

1 Webster (1995).
2 Trillat (1986, p. 274).
3 Tarde (1969).
4 Foucault (1989, p. 33).
5 Verhaeghe (1996, p. 83).
6 Deleuze (2005, p. 46).
7 Showalter (1997).
8 Deleuze (2004, p. xix).
9 In this context, Sadie Plant of the British Cybernetic Culture Research Unit uses the term *hyperstitions*, a blend of the words *hype* and *superstition*. *Hyperstitions* are fictions that retroactively create the conditions that allow them to become reality.

Chapter 2

The fathers of hysteria

Introduction

The 19th century got off to a hysterical start. An unprecedented fierceness and determination radiated from people, as if they were possessed by the rage of a much larger person. They seemed to be more irritable, quicker to get annoyed at small things and to react with exaggerated vehemence to setbacks and adversity. A satisfactory explanation for this behaviour was not found until the second half of the 19th century, when hysteria took on epidemic proportions and physicians started studying the condition intensely in specially designated and equipped hospital wards. The epidemic would last for almost three decades and cast a shadow on the glamour and glitter of the 1878 Paris World's Fair, intended as a celebration of the reconstruction of France after the war with Germany. While this was a relatively short period, it is still referred to as the golden age of hysteria.

In the 19th century, hysteria broke out all over Europe, in rural areas as well as in the big cities. The illness spread especially fast in France and Germany; as far as it is possible to ascertain, Paris counted over 50,000 female hysteria sufferers aged between 13 and 35 at the end of the 19th century. With hysteria spreading so quickly, hysterics were locked up and treated in hospitals like the Hôpital de la Salpêtrière in Paris, which originally dated from the 17th century and was the leading mental health institution of the time. In 1880, almost a quarter of women admitted to this medical centre, run by physician Jean-Martin Charcot, were diagnosed with hysteria, compared with just 1% in the 1840s. Academic publications on the condition also increased conspicuously. Between 1880 and 1900, over 130 papers on hysteria were published in France alone, with such magnificent titles as *Les hystériques: État physique et état mental* (1883), *Les maladies de la personnalité* (1885) and *Une observation de grande hystérie chez l'homme* (1886).

But as quickly as hysteria had appeared, it vanished again. Around 1893, hospitals had hardly any hysterical patients left on their wards, and you rarely encountered hysterical people in the street. Thirty years of hysteria had come to an end, but the illness's disappearance still raised many questions. Why had it vanished so suddenly? What had caused the epidemic in the first place? The answer to these questions is neither easy to grasp nor to summarise. The emergence and disappearance of hysteria can be explained on a relatively short time scale, as well as in the context of a larger historical development. Before I go into the *belle époque* of hysteria in more detail, I would like to take a look at that broader picture. Hysteria has been known since ancient Egyptian times, where it was thought to be an illness that caused the womb to wander through the body.

In an attempt to shed a little light on the history of hysteria, I will show the different approaches that have been taken to understanding the illness, variously as a somatic, a supernatural and a psychological phenomenon. What makes these perspectives remarkable is their link to specific physical configurations, which range from the womb and the stake to the psychiatric clinic and the psychiatrist's couch.

The wandering womb

The womb is our very first living space, our first home, as it were. Our first experiences take place in its intimate comfort and safety, where bodily substances are exchanged between mother and child through the umbilical cord. The moment the infant is forced to leave the peaceful womb that has been its home for so long, and is severed, screaming, from the umbilical cord, it enters the precarious outside world. It will continue to seek the protection of new spaces in order to relive the homelike feeling of the womb and the sense of comfort and security it offered, such as huts, houses, villages, tribes, companies, neighbourhoods and nation states. This is why the German philosopher Peter Sloterdijk believes that all of the world's other 'spheres' are modelled on the womb, or uterus, and that society can be viewed as a 'utero-technical project', in which humans are constantly trying to wall or fence themselves in.[1]

In his monumental magnum opus *Spheres*, a 2500-page reflection on the uterus's protective function, Sloterdijk examines the numerous spaces in which humans develop into humans, starting with the small world of the uterus. He repeatedly shows that we go in search of new spaces to relive our early experience in the womb, in an effort to compensate for the lost uterine one-ness. Sloterdijk illustrates his basic idea by quoting a passage from the 1977 book *L'oreille et la vie* by the French physician Alfred Tomatis, who developed listening therapies for people with voice problems and difficulties learning and communicating:

> The mother will always be this magnified uterus, this face that later becomes a hut, an igloo, a house, the universe. We are always surrounded by walls. We never truly leave the uterus, though it expands in the course of our lives, taking on other forms and proportions.[2]

Reading Sloterdijk's *Spheres*, it is difficult to avoid the conclusion that his spatial anthropology is ontologically anchored in the womb, the place that offers the child safe and comfortable protection against the big bad outside world. At the same time, there is a darker side to his theory, one that does not even get a mention in his whole trilogy about 'spheres', 'bubbles' and 'foam'. I am referring to the traditional meaning of the word 'hysteria', as an illness of the womb. The word comes from the Ancient Greek ὑστερικός and the Latin *hystericus*, which means 'pertaining to the uterus' and is derived from *hustera*, womb. It is based on the belief that hysteria is caused by the womb travelling through the body, triggering a host of different symptoms on its way. According to this view, symptoms of hysteria occur when the shifting womb puts pressure on the body's organs.

The idea of the womb going astray dates back to the ancient Egyptians. In one of the oldest pieces of medical writing in existence, a papyrus from Kahun dating from around 1900 BCE, all female medical complaints are attributed to a wandering womb. The same reasoning is found in Plato's *Timaeus*, dating from around 360 BCE, in which he compares the womb to an animal that desires to bear children, a living creature with a will and desires of its own. Later, he writes:

> And if it [i.e. the womb] is left unfertilized long beyond the normal time, it causes extreme unrest, strays about the body, blocks the channels of the breath and causes in consequence acute distress and disorders of all kinds.[3]

The hungrier the womb is, the more it roams around in a woman's body. On Mondays, the womb is thought to settle in the throat, cutting off the air supply. This is also referred to as the globus hystericus – a spherical cramp that rises up from the sufferer's belly and makes the sufferer feel as if she had a lump in her throat. On Tuesdays, it latches onto the heart, causing nausea and vomiting; on Wednesdays it picks on the liver, making the woman lose her voice and grind her teeth, and turning her face ashen; and on Thursdays it is inside the head, resulting in headaches and pain around the eyes.

Devils and demons

Hysteria has traditionally been viewed as a female problem, caused by the womb wandering around in the body. The various explanations that have been found for this extraordinary behaviour of the organ are too diverse and numerous to list in their entirety, but two of them have made regular appearances throughout history: a natural and a supernatural one. The natural explanation looked for the cause of the illness in the female body, where unfulfilled sexual desires were thought to make the womb wander. Driven by its sexual urges, the hungry womb goes in search of food in the form of sperm. As a proof, proponents of this theory pointed to the fact that widows and unmarried women who were not sexually active were disproportionally prone to the illness – convents, where nuns did nothing but pray, meditate and fast, saw veritable epidemics of hysteria.

Another natural explanation of hysteria is the humoral doctrine devised by the Greek physician Hippocrates (approx. 460–370 BCE) and the Greek-Roman doctor Galenus (129–199 CE). It is based on the theory that the human body consists of four kinds of fluids – blood, black bile, yellow bile and phlegm – which correspond with the four elements fire, water, earth and air, and whose relative proportions result in certain character traits and medical conditions in people. Someone with too much black bile is melancholic and suffers from depressive disorders, while too much phlegm leads to over-sensitivity. Humourism is based on the belief that there should be a balance between the four fluids, or humours. If they get out of balance, the humour of which there is a surplus in the body should be drained.

In order for hysteria to be cured, the womb must return to its natural place. The numerous ways of achieving this are all of a highly sexual nature. Hippocrates advised women suffering from hysteria attacks to moisten the womb in order to keep it from getting dehydrated, preferably by having sex. Consequently, young girls were advised to marry or give birth. In *Een verhandeling over hypochondrische en hysterische ziekten* (A Treatise on Hypochondriac and Hysterical Diseases) from 1711, the Dutch-English physician and philosopher Bernard Mandeville prescribes daily horse riding for hysterical girls, followed by three-hour massages. The French *Manuel de médecine pratique* from 1800 contains more practical tips designed to make an end to the womb's wanderings through the body. It suggests letting the patient sniff the smell of singed leather, or pouring bitter fluids into her mouth, to encourage the womb to return to its place. Another method was to pull out some of her pubic hairs with a strong, unexpected jolt, while loudly banging on drums and shields to startle the womb and chase it back to the place it belongs. Other treatments of the time included applying leeches to the vagina and the cervix. At the end of the 19th century, female hysteria sufferers were even treated with vibrators powered by spring mechanisms, as seen in the 2011 movie *Hysteria* about the physicians Joseph Mortimer Granville and Robert Dalrymple, who treated women for hysteria in Victorian England.

The natural explanation focused on hysteria as a medical problem, a view that changed in the course of the Middle Ages, when hysteria was increasingly considered a moral problem. Women suffering from a serious form of hysteria were thought to be possessed by devils and demons. Hysterical women were no longer ill, but the victims – or worse, handmaidens – of the devil. Their bodies were possessed by some evil demon as a punishment for committing sins. The vagina being an open door for the devil, women ran a greater risk of being possessed than men; a view that was in fact still a blend of natural and supernatural explanations. Around 400 CE, the church father Augustine of Hippo still believed that hysteria had everything to do with a woman's need for sex, but instead of attributing her insatiable libido to the womb, he now claimed it was the work of the devil. In *Malleus maleficarum*, the 1487 treatise on witchcraft colloquially know as the *Hammer of Witches*, hysterics are described as being tools of the devil in his battle against Christianity. While the main theme of *Malleus maleficarum* is witchcraft, hysteria is never far away in this book. Its authors Heinrich Kramer and Jacob Sprenger write that 'many, if not all, witches are hysterics, as are a large part of their victims'. Kramer was born in Schlettstadt, a town to the south-east of Strasbourg, in 1430. At a very early age, he entered the Dominican order (the 'Dogs of God'), established by the Church to keep believers from straying. Originally from Basle, Sprenger was appointed dean of the Faculty of Theology at the University of Cologne. Their book *Malleus maleficarum* became the ultimate handbook and undisputed authority for witch hunters such as the inquisition, judges and Catholic priests. With thirteen reprints between 1487 and 1520, the book turned into a veritable bestseller. In recognition of their knowledge, the two authors were appointed Inquisitors by Pope Innocent VIII and charged with investigating crimes of witchcraft in northern Germany.

Hysterics suspected of witchcraft were sentenced to death for collaborating with the devil and his demons. Women were the main targets. Between the 15th and early 18th centuries, over 100,000 people were subjected to witch trials in Europe, and about half of that number were sentenced to death. The intensity of witch hunts peaked in France and Switzerland in the first half of the 17th century, and in Germany during the Thirty Years' War (1618–1648). But people were burnt at the stake in other parts of Europe as well. It is estimated that a total of between 30,000 and 60,000 Europeans were put to death for allegedly making a pact with the devil, and that about 80% of them were women.

Clouded brain

Because the womb symbolises the essence of a woman's body, hysteria has always been considered a typically female phenomenon. It is a *mal de mère*, an illness that affects mainly women, and the restless female temper and constant mood swings that are thought to be indicative of a hysterical temperament conjure up images of the highly strung and exceptionally emotional woman. In an article in the Dutch *Tijdschrift voor psychiatrie* (Journal of Psychiatry), Frans Gilson provides a summary of the most important typologies of women suffering from hysteria in the 19th century.[4] One of them is the *femme fragile*, a pitiable, hard-working woman whose life has been a failure and who is exceptionally prone to hysteria. In the arts, the femme fragile is associated with the plant kingdom. Paintings often depict her as a flower, emphasising her fragile personality. Then there is the *femme fatale*, an alluring woman who lies and cheats and has close ties with the devil. Associated with the animal kingdom, the femme fatale is often depicted in the company of snakes, to illustrate her unpredictable personality and erratic behaviour. Finally, there is the *femme savante*, a learned woman who wants to be treated equally to men. The *femme savante* is above all an object of pity. Nineteenth-century women were expected to be caring housewives, and while personal development was not forbidden, it was only appreciated if the acquired knowledge was used to run the household.

In the 17th century, physicians like Charles le Pois, Thomas Willis and Thomas Sydenham first report on cases of hysteria appearing in men. Before that time, men with hysterical symptoms were diagnosed as hypochondriacs. This change of view was caused by the discovery of anatomists that the womb is not in fact able to move around in the body, which also put an end to the notion of the womb as a hungry animal causing hysteria in a patient, and ushered in the search for other causes of the illness. Le Pois, founder of the medical faculty at Pont-à-Mousson University in the Lotharingen region, studied the brain for an explanation of hysteria, concluding that the brain is confused by an imbalance of bodily fluids caused by intense passions. According to his theory, the fluids enter the brain and cloud the mind. Thomas Sydenham, a kind of English Hippocrates, also searched for the cause of hysteria in the human mind. He believed in 'animal spirits' (*spiritus animales*) located in the brain and nervous system that go out of control and independently carry out tasks in other parts of the body. Today, we would call these animal spirits electric impulses in the nervous system. According to Sydenham, the bodily functions are impaired by such 'confused spirits', which interfere with bodily functions that should be controlled by other spirits, causing confusion in the brain. Sydenham calls this process 'an incorrect distribution of animal spirits in the system'.

Despite the growing body of evidence in the 17th century that the womb plays no part in the occurrence of hysteria, it took another two centuries before the ancient uterus theories were definitely shelved, and before the possibility of hysteria affecting men as well as women was seriously considered. Even then, it did not happen without a struggle. As late as 1819, the French physician Jean-Baptiste Louyer-Villermay claimed that 'a man cannot be hysterical, as he does not have a womb'. In his 1846 *Traité complet de l'hystérie*, Hector Landouzy writes that hysteria is caused by 'disorders of the womb or ovaries',[5] and in 1883, the French physician Augustin Fabre argues in *L'hystérie viscérale* that all women are hysterical and every woman 'carries the seeds of hysteria with her'. As it turned out, a large majority of patients labelled as hysterical were in fact female.[6] In the Netherlands between 1875 and 1900, many more hysterical women than men were institutionalised – 1340 women compared with 116 men, to be precise.[7] The reason for this is that men were less likely to be diagnosed with hysteria because they were thought to be far less prone to the disease, with the exception of homosexuals, Jews and tramps. Colloquially, hysteria continued to be known as a 'female disease', diagnosed by 'male doctors'. One of the best known of these male doctors is the previously mentioned Jean-Martin Charcot, professor of pathological anatomy and neurology in Paris.

Charcot's theatre

Charcot was born in Paris in 1825 and began his medical studies in 1843. In 1862, he became a physician at the Salpêtrière hospital in Paris, an enormous medical complex that consisted of 45 buildings, roads, squares, gardens and its own church. The hospital was named after the former gunpowder factory that is part of the complex, the Petit Arsenal-Salpêtrière. In 1656, the factory was converted into a refuge for the poor and the handicapped. As a part of l'Hospice Général, it was dedicated to women and girls, and not much later, the Salpêtrière became the foremost medical centre in Europe for the housing and treatment of hysterics. Charcot called the Salpêtrière a 'living museum of pathology'. In 1870, one of the buildings in the complex became so derelict that its inhabitants, primarily epileptics and hysterics, were all moved into the Quartier des épileptiques simples, which was under Charcot's direction. This set in motion his study into hysteria, and a decade later, he had become the leading authority in France and abroad in the fields of hysteria and hypnosis.

Charcot's work was descriptive at first, carefully observing and describing his hysterical patients' behavioural patterns and subdividing the condition into separate, consecutive stages. With this approach, Charcot wanted to make a clear division between the symptoms of hysteria and those of other illnesses, and to create a point of departure for a better understanding of the condition. While basing his research mostly on his patients at Salpêtrière, Charcot writes in an 1882 issue of Le progrès médical that hysteria 'is a timeless phenomenon and occurs in all countries, people, religions and races'. According to Charcot, hysteria itself is not only universal, but attacks of la grande hystérie always follow a similar pattern. He believed that hysteria has a fixed course that can be divided into four phases. The first phase is heralded by an aching sensation in the area around the ovaries. This 'epileptoid phase' is characterised by cramps and later spasms, during which the patient flails around wildly, pulls out their hair and tears off their clothes. In the second, even more spectacular phase that is sometimes called 'clownism', the patient twists their body and makes other grands mouvements such as the well-known arc-en-ciel, in which the body becomes as bent as a hoop, only resting on the back of the head and the heels. The third phase is marked by impassioned movements such as taking up a praying position, standing like a cross or striking erotically charged poses. Charcot links this 'hallucinatory phase' to religious ecstasy. The fourth and last phase, the 'terminal delusion', is a final delirium (délire). The patient's experience of this can vary greatly, ranging from hallucinations to revelations from their past.

In 1878, Charcot first examined patients using electronic devices, shifting his methodology from clinical observation to physiological research.[8] He studied hysteria with the use of metal and magnets, and used hypnosis on his patients. He also made more intensive use than before of drawings and photographs in order to document the symptoms of hysteria as comprehensively as possible, regarding the photographs he took of hysterical patients as an 'objective record' of the illness. They were printed in the *Iconographie photographique de la Salpê-trière* journal, published between 1875 and 1880. In 1882, he writes that 'our research into hysteria will bring us honour and glory, and the French school will triumph around the world'. But despite the meticulous study of his patients, Charcot failed to discover an overarching theory of the cause of hysteria. He attempted to explain the illness mainly by combining various insights of other physicians. For example, he traced the cause of hysteria to a combination of physical defects (*tare nerveuse*) located in the cerebral cortex, with possible reflectory effects from the ovaries, and short-term triggers (*agents provocateurs*) such as alcoholism and trauma. Other physicians before him had already located hysteria in the brain, caused by a traumatic injury or heredi-tary defect in the patient's nervous system, and echoes of this theory can be found in the work of the above-mentioned Le Pois and Sydenham. Charcot believed the aetiology of hysteria lay in heredity, according to the doctrine of the *famille névropathique*, and that it followed the female line. He was not alone in this opinion, either – many physicians before him believed that hereditary degeneration played a key role in the development of hysteria.

The most important point for the subject of this chapter is that with Charcot, hysteria shifted from the stake to the hospital. Instead of being publicly executed on suspicion of being in league with the devil, hysterical women were locked up in psychiatric institutions. You could say that burning at the stake gave way to observation, diagnosis and treatment. It should be noted that the term observa-tion is used in its broadest sense here, as the Salpêtrière was far more than just a hospital. Among other things, the complex comprised an amphitheatre with four hundred seats in which Charcot held weekly lectures on hysteria, and where he examined hysterical patients on a platform in the middle of the room. He used his Tuesday lectures to present his findings in the field of hysteria like a true performing artist, and the papers reported widely on his theatrical performances. In such public displays of its poses and positions, the hysterical body became synonymous with a fundamental theatricality, echoes of which still reverberate in everyday language about hysteria today. It was this theatricalisation of the hys-terical body that prompted Georges Didi-Huberman's comparison to a work of art in his 1982 book *Invention de l'hystérie.*[9] Charcots performances, which lasted two hours on average, were extremely popular for their high entertainment value. Besides leading physicians like Pierre Janet, William James and Sigmund Freud, his lectures also attracted large numbers of non-medical professionals like journalists, artists, writers, actresses and politicians. Charcot's performances were a forerunner of Antonin Artaud's theatrical work, described by Artaud in his 1927 essay 'Manifesto for a Theatre That Failed' as the 'authentic performance of magic', Fluxus art events, and rock concerts by such bands as Einstürzende Neubauten.

Charcot's fame spread throughout France, especially when the number of hysterics and patients suffering from hysterical symptoms started rising specta-cularly in the late 1870s. The fact that this was the very period in which

Charcot started to focus on hysteria is certainly no coincidence. It was rumoured that Charcot attributed everything that was 'not right' about the body or mind to hysteria, claiming that sleep and even death could be hysterical. As a result in 1880, almost a quarter of all patients at the Salpêtrière hospital were diagnosed with hysteria. Statistics show that in the middle of the 1880s, 20% of all patients were labelled hysterical, while this percentage was only 1% in the 1840s. The proportion of hysterics subsequently dropped to 10% in 1888 and to 6% in 1894, a year after Charcot died of a heart attack on holiday in de Morvan.[10] After his death, the number of hysterical patients at Salpêtrière and in other parts of the world dropped still further, and it was not long before there were no more hysterical patients in hospitals at all. The universal laws of hysteria that Charcot had 'discovered' faded from prominence and were forgotten. The illness vanished completely.

On Freud's couch

It was Sigmund Freud, the founding father of psychoanalysis, who breathed new life into hysteria. His ideas on the influence of the subconscious and the constant struggle between the life and death drives were crucial in forming the self-image of the 20th-century public. In October 1885, the 29-year-old Freud moved to Paris, where he became Charcot's pupil until the middle of 1886. He was so impressed by Charcot's teaching and work that he translated two of his books, *Leçons sur les maladies du système nerveux* and *Leçons de mardi*, into German. In gratitude for the translation, Charcot gave Freud a leather-bound edition of his collected works with the inscription 'A Monsieur le Docteur Freud, excellents souvenirs de la Salpêtrière – Charcot'. Freud later named his first-born son Jean-Martin. Freud initially adhered to Charcot's conclusion that the cause for hysteria could be found in the brain, and that genetics played a large part in its emergence. In 1888, Freud writes that 'The aetiology of the status hystericus is to be looked for entirely in heredity; hysterics are always hereditarily disposed to disturbances of nervous activity, and epileptics, psychical patients, tabetics, etc. are found among their relatives.'[11]

But despite admiring Charcot's work, Freud gradually broke free from the views on the causes of hysteria that had prevailed until then. He did not share the notion of the womb as a living creature, or in his own words, a 'dark beast', and eventually, Charcot's ideas on the brain and the heredity of hysteria also lost their appeal for him. Instead, Freud searched for the cause of hysteria elsewhere, viewing the illness as a psychological or subconscious conflict that finds a physical outlet in hysterical attacks. He described this process as the repression of unpleasant memories and inappropriate thoughts rooted in traumatic, often sexual, experiences, which are subsequently expressed through physical symptoms such as partial paralysis and extreme stiffness, reduced appetite, bizarre gait pattern, mood swings, retching and vomiting, coughing, headache, depression, insomnia and speech impediments. In a talk to the Viennese Psychiatric Society on 21

April 1896 titled 'On the Aetiology of Hysteria', Freud explained that traumas function as 'symbols of memory' and that their most striking trait is that they cannot be put into words, which makes a normal healing process impossible. Freud and the general practitioner Josef Breuer referred to this by the term 'conversion', a phenomenon of body language. In *Studien über Hysterie*, they describe trauma as 'any experience that gives rise to the painful affects of fright, fear, shame or physical pain, taking into account that it depends on the sensitivity of the person whether or not the experience is traumatising'.[12]

Freud and Breuer's analysis of conversion shows that the underlying trauma does not actually need to have taken place – as they show in *Studien über Hysterie*, it can also be a fantasy or a forbidden desire. Alternatively, the cause can be a series of traumas and the fantasies connected to them, which can be traced back to their origin in therapy. This is illustrated by the first case study described in *Studien über Hysterie,* the case history of Anna O., who was later identified as the Austrian Jew Bertha Pappenheim. Breuer treated Anna in his office in Vienna between November 1880 and July 1882. The 20-year-old suffered from hysterical symptoms including paraphrasia, loss of sight and paralysis of her arm and both legs, and Breuer cured her of her hysterical attacks by making her relive traumatic experiences under hypnosis. One such experience had left her unable to drink a glass of water, eating fruit such as melons to quench her thirst. She told Breuer under hypnosis that she had once seen the dog of her English lady companion drink out of a water glass and felt deeply disgusted, but had been too polite to tell the woman off at the time. Still under hypnosis, she then asked Breuer for a glass of water and drank from it, eventually waking from her hypnosis with the glass still at her lips. Breuer managed to find other traumatic experiences in Anna's past and made her relive them under hypnosis, at which they disappeared and she was cured of hysteria.

In October 1900, Freud discovered the same conversion of mental stimuli into hysterical symptoms in the 18-year-old Dora, whom he treated in his office on 19 Berggasse in Vienna, only a few streets away from the university. This was the place where Freud searched the psyches of his patients like a private investigator in order to unravel the mystery of hysteria, though he was not so much interested in the classic question of 'whodunit' but rather 'whydunit', i.e., why people become hysterical. Freud's famous couch, the place where Dora gave her thoughts free rein in free association, is not just another sofa. It is a horsehair chaise longue covered by a woven red Persian rug and a large variety of cushions, and flanked on either side by Egyptian, Roman and Greek artefacts that Freud had collected on his many travels. Freud's dark green armchair was placed behind the head of the couch because he did not want his patients to constantly stare at him. The Russian aristocrat Sergei Pankejeff, one of Freud's most famous patients who became known as the Wolf Man, describes the atmosphere in Freud's office as follows:

> There was always a feeling of sacred peace and quiet here. The rooms themselves must have been a surprise to any patient, for they in no way

reminded one of a doctor's office but rather of an archaeologist's study. [...] Everything here contributed to one's feeling of leaving the haste of modern life behind, of being sheltered from one's daily cares.[13]

At first, Freud wanted to give Dora's case history the title *Traum und Hysterie*, but later changed it to *Bruchstück einer Hysterie-Analyse*. While this case study is not a systematic analysis of the nature of hysteria, it does include an excellent description of it. Dora suffered from many different forms of 'minor hysteria', a less spectacular form of hysteria that includes shortness of breath, nervous coughing, loss of voice and a constant tendency to quarrel. Tracing back a network of interacting traumas during the sessions, Freud discovered Dora's infatuation with Mr K, the husband of the woman Dora's father was having an affair with. This Mr K had declared Dora his love during a walk following a boat trip on the lake, and this event reminded Dora of a trauma that had taken place years earlier, when Mr K pulled the 14-year-old Dora close to him in his shop and kissed her on the lips. Freud noted that Dora could feel K's erection pressing against her body during the embrace. Instead of sexual arousal – Freud points out that Mr K is a youthful man with a pleasant appearance – Dora only felt a deep repulsion, and ran out of the door. Freud writes:

> I should without question consider a person hysterical in whom an occasion for sexual excitement elicited feelings that were preponderantly or exclusively unpleasurable; and I should do so whether or not the person were capable of producing somatic symptoms.[14]

In his analysis of Dora, Freud argues that her hysterical complaints stem from her guilty feelings about her sexual attraction to Mr K. Without using the term 'Oedipus complex', Freud discovered the Oedipal theme in Dora's desire for her father's affection and her wish to give her father that which her mother denied him.

After Dora, Freud's work focused mainly on boys ('Little Hans') and men ('the Rat Man'), and hysteria moved to the background to make way for two other psychoneuroses: paranoia and compulsive-obsessive neurosis. In spite of that, he continues to address hysteria in his work with some regularity, though it is not always entirely clear how Freud meant to approach the condition. There is a constant change of emphasis, with Freud initially claiming that passive sexual experiences in early childhood lead to hysteria, and active experiences to compulsive obsessive neurosis. He also believed that the form the neurosis takes is influenced by the stage of life in which the trauma took place, or, according to yet another insight, by the stage of life in which defence mechanisms against reliving the traumatic experience are developed. In 'Three Essays on the Theory of Sexuality' from 1905, he focuses on the relationship between 'an immense sexual desire on the one hand and a highly exaggerated sexual rejection on the other'.[15] This divides the concept of hysteria into a sexual component, repression in the form of defence ('not knowing'), and the manifestation of suppressed feelings as physical symptoms. Contrarily, in 'The Disposition of Obsessional Neurosis' from 1913, Freud searches for an explanation in the various problems the neuroses present, which he believed correspond with the nature of what he called their 'dispositions'. He was hoping to find an answer to the question of why a person suffered from one kind of neurosis and not another. Why, for instance, did someone become hysterical and not paranoid? Freud came to believe that a person could be hysterical even before suffering traumas. According to him, a person's disposition determines which events are experienced as traumatic, while traumas simultaneously activate a pre-existing disposition.

I will not examine the question whether Freud found a conclusive explanation of hysteria any further. What is relevant, is that Freud's method of treating hysteria – in which the patient speaks to a psychiatrist – was comparatively new. Instead of observing his patients, Freud subjected them to a talking cure. You could also summarise the difference between his approach and that of his French mentor as follows: Charcot watched, while Freud listened. The action took place in a dimly lit room, in which the patient lay on a couch that exuded an Eastern voluptuousness. In daily sessions, Freud spent hours listening to the detailed complaints of his predominantly female patients. Examining each complaint meticulously, Freud based his thesis on the psychological causes of hysteria – of which he considered trauma to be the most important – on those conversations. He believed that physical symptoms usually ascribed to organic causes actually had a psychological origin, and that consequently, hysteria and all its associated symptoms should no longer be considered a deliberately feigned illness aimed at attracting the attention of other people. On the contrary, he argued they should be regarded as a medium for communicating a message that, for a host of reasons, could not be conveyed in any other way. Robert Woolsey called this a 'protolanguage', a unique code a person uses to express themselves.[16] In other words, hysteria and its bodily symptoms point the therapist to deeper traumas that would otherwise have been missed. By trying to fathom hysteria, the traumas are discovered. Those are key points to understanding hysteria in our society today. There is, however, another approach, developed by Michel Foucault.

An ideological concept

Despite Charcot and Freud's widely divergent approaches to uncovering the cause of hysteria, Foucault gives both of them a central role in his 1976 book *The Will to Knowledge*. Among other things, Foucault points out that Freud unmasking Dora's desire as an Oedipus complex coincided with the period in which a law was passed to criminalise incest. At the same moment, in other words, that psychoanalysis brought a desire for incest to light, it was made punishable by law. Foucault calls Charcot's hospital 'an enormous apparatus for observation, with its examinations, interrogations, and experiments'.[17] He considers Freud's practice of confession and Charcot's lecture theatre as benchmarks, because they use hysteria as a starting point in the search of the truth about human nature. In line with Nietzsche's analysis of truth and lies, he argues that truth is not something that is discovered, but rather constructed or invented. Put another way, truth does not exist but was created in a discourse on sex and sexuality that originated in the late 18th century. Foucault treats sex and sexuality as collective terms for 'the set of effects produced in bodies, behaviours, and social relations by a certain deployment deriving from a complex political technology'.[18] According to him, this sexual discourse provides the framework in which the speaking and acting on sex and sexuality take place. He does not, however, view all this talk about sex and sexuality as a sign of greater freedom – on the contrary, the more sex is discussed, the more precisely can all its aspects and characteristics be mapped. This not only means that our knowledge of sex is still growing, which has the added benefit of making it easier to analyse and explain, but more importantly, that it becomes easier to control. To this end, a veritable apparatus has been put in place which permanently monitors our sexuality in the name of truth and normality.

Foucault identified four deviant identities that strongly colour the debate on sex, each of which sets the norm for their positive opposite: the masturbating child, the perverse adult, the non-reproductive married couple and the hysterical woman. Despite the great differences of these four categories, they are similar in that they become the product of a specific kind of knowledge and power (a power that is knowledge and a knowledge that is power), which runs through the family and which is placed under supervision and surveillance. Foucault writes that the family is 'the crystal in the deployment of sexuality: it seemed to be the source of a sexuality which it actually only reflected and diffracted'.[19] According to him, a woman's body is hystericalised in three separate processes. First of all, her body is analysed and qualified, only to be disqualified as being ill and abnormal. Simultaneously, the pathology inherent to this means the hysterical woman is admitted into the practice of the medical world. In this process, the body of the woman is inextricably linked to the body of society, whose fertility she must regulate and guaranteed by bearing and raising children. and everything is done in the name of woman's responsibility for the health of her children, the stability of the family and the welfare of society.

Foucault's major contribution to a better understanding of hysteria is the fact that in each of these three processes, disciplinary techniques are accompanied by regulatory mechanisms. On the one hand, the hysterical woman gives rise to the need for meticulous forms of supervision and constant monitoring through endless medical and psychological examinations, while on the other, her wider effects on the well-being of society lead to measurements on a national level, statistical estimations and interventions in the societal body as a whole or in separate groups. Against this background, hysteria becomes a political undertaking that falls under the administration of the government. This means that the analysis of hysteria is no longer focused on sin and run by the institution of the church, but takes place in the institution of the nation state and scientific disciplines such as demography (coordinated birth campaigns), pedagogics (child sexuality) and medicine (sexual physiology of women). Hysteria has left the Christian domain of death and eternal punishment to become a problem of life and illness.

In his article 'La politique de la santé au XVIIIe siècle', Foucault coined the term *nosopolitique* to interpret the interaction of diseases, the people suffering from them, medical science and politics.[20] *Nosos* is an ancient Greece word for 'disease'. Nosopolitics, a variation of biopolitics, focuses on controlling the conditions that influence public health, such as introducing birth control and bringing down child mortality. The duties of the police force are a good example of this policy, as they consist not only of fighting crime and disorder but also of monitoring compliance with numerous hygiene rules, such as the removal of litter from the streets, inspection of food sold in markets, ventilation of buildings, and so on. By focusing their efforts on the immediate surroundings of citizens, the police attempt to change them in order to improve quality of life. Physicians, pedagogues and psychiatrists also focus on more than just treating patients. They educate the public about healthy dietary habits and advise families on the upbringing of babies and toddlers, besides holding important positions in well-known breeding grounds of disease such as prisons, ships and shelters for homeless people and beggars. The aim of this all is to make life stronger and more resilient, and therefore increasing the productivity of citizens and the prosperity of society. Foucault correctly remarks that this means hysteria is not just a medical issue but also a social and political problem. A hysteria diagnosis becomes an ideologically determined concept, a tool to discipline and organise society and others.

An unattainable desire

Freud's analyses have set many an academic pen in motion, and much has been written about how Freud's numerous publications lay the foundations for psychoanalysis, about his extensive case studies of hysterical patients such as Anna O., Dora and Cäcilie M., his accounts of the Wolf Man's dreams, and how he seemed to trace everything back to the Oedipus complex. Even if most of Freud's interpretations did not stand the test of time and he was maligned for some of his more misogynist conclusions (such as his remarks in the Dora case on the attraction Mr K exerted on young women), we are indebted to him for the realisation that desire plays an important part in explaining human behaviour. This desire, which Freud often believed to be of a sexual nature, exists in the subconscious until it is replaced by some form of satisfaction. As Freud's analyses of his hysterical patients show, however, the problem with this is that satisfaction is very rarely permanent. Why else would Freud's patients keep reliving their traumas, in the guise of countless fragmentary experiences?

This is the question Jacques Lacan explored further in the weekly seminars he gave in Paris in the 1950s and 1960s, taking the next step towards a better understanding of hysteria. But while Lacan claimed to be 'returning to Freud', their analyses differed considerably. Rather than an unquestioning repetition, his return was fuelled by new insights in the field of psychology and inspired by developments in other scientific fields, including linguistics and anthropology. One important difference is that Lacan's analysis is based not on the libido but on the structure of language. In his early seminars, Lacan argued that humans are constructed by language. As speaking beings ('*Ça parle!*'), Lacan writes that we need language to get a hold on something, such as for instance the subconscious. Entering the order of language has the unpleasant consequence that the immediate experience of daily life is lost, making humans feel a permanent sense of lack, and consequently an unattainable desire (*le désir*). Following in Freud's footsteps, Lacan believed that this unattainable desire, fundamental to all humans, is where the essence of hysteria lies. He calls the structure of this desire hysterical.

Lacan did not view hysteria as a nosological category, but in a metonymic sense, that is to say that the desire of women as well as men shifts continuously. There is no final endpoint because it constantly changes focus. You could also say that the endpoint of desire is imaginary. For this reason, the essence or the nature of desire, and with it of hysteria, can never be defined or grasped. Desire escapes every attempt at definition because its contents are constantly changing. Lacan calls the object of desire the 'object a', emphasising the difference between cause and object of desire, and pointing to the fact that any object capable of satisfying desire leads to a new lack, which in turn generates more desire. This lack, which is constantly recreated and which lies at the basis of desire, is insatiable. Lacan calls this lack, this chasm between the world and us, our desires and the meanings we assign to the world, a 'lack of being'. Since we never really succeed in filling this lack, it becomes a structural part of human existence.

A quick online search yields plenty of examples of this never-sated desire. Take the popularity of consumer articles such as the telephone, which currently passes as 'smart'. The launch of every new iPhone sends us running to Apple Stores in a crazed frenzy, even though everyone knows the difference between the old and new versions is small and in no way justifies the expensive purchase. And yet we feel we are missing out unless we replace our old smart phone with the latest model. Eyes glued to the screen of our new iPhone, we are then confronted with the world around us and with such problems as the refugee and climate crises, which are so vast and abstract they go beyond the human imagination. At the same time, the cause of our desire is already driving us towards the next iPhone model. The same thing happens with everything else, all the time, every day.

To really understand what makes us into such hysterical creatures, Lacan makes an illuminating distinction between demand (*la demande*) and need (*le besoin*). In Lacan's view, demand always takes place on a conscious level; as human beings, we are only able to express ourselves through demands. But the demand is far more than a simple demand: it is based on a need. This need is of a physiological nature and often concerns such purely vital necessities as food and drink, in which case it is always aimed at a certain object that can satisfy the need. When I feel the need of a glass of wine, I can crack open a bottle of Bourgogne to quench my thirst. Lacan adds to this that my desire always underpins my need and always exceeds it. But while desire itself also pursues a certain object, no single concrete object can satisfy it because it does not have a definitive end point – it is always the desire for more, for something that can never fully be achieved.

The difference between demand, need and desire is crucial to Lacan because without this distinction, humans would be one with the satisfaction of their basic needs. In other words, denying the existence of desire is reducing human life to a purely animal existence. Without desire, humans would lose their zest for living. What is more, since desire keeps shifting, Lacan argues that the desire of a hysterical subject consists of having an unfulfilled desire. Attempts to discuss this desire are doomed to failure, since it can never completely be expressed in language – unlike demand, desire takes place on a subconscious level. It is unable to explain what makes the desired object so meaningful, which is why a person never knows exactly what it is they desire. What do they really want? The impossibility of putting the desire into words also pertains to the relationship between the desire and its object – as is shown in the example of the latest iPhone. The object can never match the desire completely, because the desire cannot express itself with perfect accuracy. This inability to express the desire results in the impossibility of making it converge with the desired object. In other words, the desire divides the subject and object, making hysteria into an intangible phenomenon. The result of this is that hysteria cannot be cured either by physicians, politicians or scientists – or in fact anyone else. This is the most important lesson to be gleaned from Lacan's work.

Conclusion

No matter how many interpretations of hysteria you come up with, one aspect of the condition presents itself immediately: hysteria is constantly appearing on and disappearing from the world stage. Throughout its long history, it has variously been explained as a somatic, a supernatural and a psychological phenomenon, but a closer look at these three explanations soon shows they cannot be neatly divided from one another. They overlap and have often been used interchangeably, as becomes evident from looking at Enlightenment era medical explanations of hysteria, which still feature devils and demons taking possession of a person's body. This is also reflected in the fact that when a woman stands up for herself too vehemently, she is still made out to be a hysterical witch – an image that dates back to medieval times. There is one thing everyone agrees on, however: as the explanations have changed, so have prevailing opinions on who should make the diagnosis, what treatment is appropriate and where the patient should be treated.

I opened this chapter with the question why hysteria vanished so suddenly at the end of the 19th century. Where did hysteria go? Explanations for this can be found in three different fields.[21] Firstly, society has become more open since the 19th century, resulting in freer morals. Compared with the suffocating Victorian era, nicknamed the 'age of chastity', women have been given more freedom to express themselves in many fields. Speaking about sex is no longer taboo, and feelings can be expressed publicly. The sexual revolution broke out as a response to the Victorian era, which incidentally affected men as well as women – for one thing, they discovered that women were driven by the same base instincts as they were. A second explanation is that under Freud's growing influence in psychology as well as outside the circle of physicians and psychiatrists, hysteria became less popular. It may sound like a paradox, but Freud's ideas generated a lot of resistance and criticism. Charcot, for example, showed little to no interest in Freud's psychology of hysteria. As Freud writes in his analysis of his patient Dora, other colleagues also rejected his insights because of the alleged 'unwarranted generalisation of conclusions' in his case studies. Put another way, for every person to say something positive about Freud, someone else could be found who considered him a scientific charlatan. Finally, with medical science developing countless new diagnoses and criteria, many symptoms of hysteria were distributed across other diagnoses. Epileptic and hysterical attacks, previously in the same category, were now divided, so that the treatment of the epileptic became completely different from that of the hysteric.

Today's medical practitioners no longer diagnose patients with hysteria. The condition has been removed from the table of contents of the DSM, the American handbook that serves as a gold standard for psychiatric diagnosis and whose 1844 predecessor first classified the inmates of mental institutions. Having said that, it is doubtful that hysteria has disappeared from society for good.[22] Today, for example, many people are extremely preoccupied about their health, and the amount of gluten in their diet in particular. Gluten, so they believe, is pure poison, fattening and terribly addictive. One in three Americans tries to avoid gluten, even though there is no medical justification for this fear whatsoever; the only reason for a gluten-free diet is coeliac disease, which only 0.3% of the population suffer from. But because of this health hysteria, all our food has to be gluten-free, and the supermarket shelves are stacked with gluten-free pasta, pizza and pancake batter. Even lollipops are labelled 'gluten-free', despite never having contained any gluten in the first place. All of this is part of the latest trend of products marketed as being 'free' of any harmful ingredients, whose popularity can be explained by the fact we are obsessed with anything that could harm us. Food is increasingly blamed for such health problems as migraine, fatigue, joint pain and other aches and pains that do not have an obvious cause. Oversimplified, it can be boiled down to the following paradox: the healthier we are objectively, the more ill we feel.

'Aren't we all a little hysterical?', asks the well-known psychiatrist Paul Julius Möbius. A question that will always provide plenty of food for discussion;

because if hysteria is a thing of the past, how come it is so ubiquitous today? For example, we have been assured for years that our country is getting ever safer – in the home, on the street, everywhere and in all sections of the population. But while there is no doubting the spectacular decrease in crime rates in Western society or the ever-shrinking number of people who sometimes feel unsafe, many people do not care about such lists with dwindling crime figures at all. The average citizen gets incredibly worked up about the remnant of insecurity in our society and responds with unprecedented vehemence to the non-committal attitude to crime that supposedly characterises this country. News items which tie in with this potential for hysteria immediately attract attention and set all the public's alarm bells ringing. How come such emotions seem increasingly to turn into hysteria, to overwhelm us, make us feel we are losing control over them? Put differently, what is at the root of security hysteria? In the next chapter, I will look for answers to this question in our tendency to use warlike language when speaking of, or acting for, our safety.

Notes

1 Sloterdijk (2003, p. 538).
2 Sloterdijk (2003, p. 545).
3 Plato (2013, pp. 98–99).
4 Gilson (2010).
5 Landouzy (1846, p. 230).
6 Interestingly, hysterical criminals are almost always young women, as Cesare Lombroso concludes in his study *L'uomo delinquente* from 1876, in which he examines the differences and similarities in the anatomies of criminal, insane and normal people. In the category of insane criminals, he differentiates between the alcoholic criminal, the imbecile criminal and the hysterical criminal. Referring to Pierre Briquet's 1859 study *Traité clinique et thérapeutique de l'hystérie*, he claims that 'hysteria [is] twenty times more frequent in women than in men' (Lombroso 2006, p. 281).
7 Schermers (1906).
8 Koehler (1995).
9 In *Totem and Taboo*, Freud takes the comparison with the arts further by saying that 'hysteria is a caricature of a work of art' (Freud 2006c, p. 84). In *La révolution sur-réaliste*, the 11th edition of the Surrealist Manifesto from 1928, Louis Aragon and André Breton, who studied medicine and psychiatry and worked on a neurological ward in the First World War, called hysteria 'the greatest poetic discovery of the late nineteenth century'.
10 Gilson (2010).
11 Freud (2006a, p. 55).
12 Freud (2006a, p. 443).
13 Pankejeff (1972, p. 139).
14 Freud (2006b, p. 143).
15 Freud (2006b, p. 46).
16 Woolsey (1976).
17 Foucault (1978, p. 55).
18 Foucault (1978, p. 127).
19 Foucault (1978, p. 111).
20 Foucault (2000, pp. 90–105).

21 Engelbrecht (2013).
22 Some authors have wondered whether the clinical picture of hysteria does not simply adapt itself to the ideas and habits prevalent in society at that moment – in other words, whether hysteria is a symptom of the spirit of the time. In her famous book *Hysteria*, Ilza Veith reasons, 'Might it not be possible that other disorders, now less clearly recognized, may be found to be aetiologically related to the complex of hysteria?' (Veith 1965, p. 10). In this regard, borderline personality disorder is considered by some to be today's equivalent of hysteria, while chronic fatigue syndrome and Gulf War syndrome also have hysterical traits.

Chapter 3

Hobbes's war

Introduction

In the past decades, our thinking about security has been dominated by a high degree of hysteria. The safer we are, the more hysterical we seem to become with regard to the remaining risk, and the consequences of this are made apparent by current security policies. All security policies are based on insecurity, and their common objective is to be tough on crime. Such policies are spoken of in terms of war, battle, struggle and survival, and with a preference for a macho military vocabulary: 'war on drugs', 'war on terror', 'war on crime', 'war on corona'. We may live in peacetime, but people are arrested by 'camouflaged and unidentified federal stormtroopers' with no explanation, your house can get raided without warning by 'intervention teams', and each year, municipalities organise a large-scale 'spring offensive' to tackle any threats to our security head-on. Security policies are designed to make clear that the days of tolerance are over and that we are locked in a fight to the death with crime and insecurity. 'Send in the troops', a Republican Senator wrote in an opinion piece in *The New York Times*, in which he advocated using the military to quell the unrest in American cities sparked by the brutal killing of George Floyd by police officers on 25 May 2020.

Hysterical use of language about security is also common in scientific writing. In his 1958 essay *Waar en waarom misdaad* (The Why and Where of Crime), Dutch criminologist Herman Bianchi writes that criminological theories sound like 'declarations of war'. Bianchi argues that the intellectually lazy and hollow military language used in criminology can be traced back to the development of an 'urge to eradicate' which started in the late 19th century, when the idea first arose that crime should be stamped out once and for all. In this respect, criminology differs considerably from such disciplines as archaeology and classical languages, which have never aimed to control or combat the subject of their studies. In fact, criminology and its belligerent language of combat and struggle has more in common with the biological and medical discourse in which everything revolves around illness, diagnosis and cure, and which similarly views its subject as a negative phenomenon that needs to be combated. This is illustrated by a statement made by French physician and criminologist Alexandre Lacassagne at the first criminological congress in Rome in 1885, barely two decades after Louis Pasteur had discovered the microbe as a pathogen, in which he compared the criminal with a microbe that can only thrive in a suitable social environment. Today, we still use medical expressions like 'prevention is better than cure' when speaking about crime.

The way security is talked about shapes our experiences of it and determines the way we handle it. Emphasising certain meanings makes them more visible, while others disappear into the background, which is why defining security in terms of warfare is not as innocent as it may seem. Language is power. Once the militant language pervades our thinking about security, 'soft' approaches to improving it are almost automatically replaced by repressive measures, even if the 'soft' approach worked better. In an effort to look decisive, policy makers pile rule upon rule, law upon law, and monitoring system upon monitoring system. In this law-enforcement pyramid, the criminal plays the part of the dangerous monster, the visible personification of everything that is evil in our society.

To get to the bottom of security hysteria we need to take a closer look at what Thomas Hobbes wrote on security. This 17th-century British thinker and his view of human nature, which he believed is dominated by evil and guided by egotism and greed, is largely responsible for our strong tendency to interpret security along the lines of such negative connotations as fear and chaos. To better understand Hobbes's deeply cynical view of mankind, we need to descend into the dark basement of the underworld, populated by all kinds of magical and monstrous creatures that personify our deepest fears. As this chapter will show, Hobbes and other thinkers viewed monstrousness as the political category par excellence for addressing the issue of security. In fact, the figure of the monster legitimises the existence of the government and the police force as crime fighting institutions – and in such circumstances, hysteria is never far behind.

The will to survive

Hobbes was born in Wiltshire in the south of England on 5 April 1588 as the son of an illiterate vicar. After beating up another vicar in a churchyard, his father fled to London, leaving his children with his brother, a glove maker. At 15 years old, Hobbes studied classics at Magdalen College, Oxford, and after graduating, got a job as a travelling companion and tutor for the family of William Cavendish, later Earl of Devonshire. Having become embroiled in a conflict between the parliament under Oliver Cromwell and the king, Hobbes fled to France in late 1640 and returned to England in 1662, constantly pursued by his political opponents. In France he wrote his first book *De Cive* (The Citizen) in 1642, and his most famous work, *Leviathan*, nine years later.

A treatise on the structure of society, *Leviathan* is considered one of the most important and influential texts in the history of philosophy. Countless thinkers of the Enlightenment either opposed it or based their own work on it. Locke, Rousseau, Beccaria, Spinoza, Kant and Leibniz, to name but a few, all engaged with Hobbes's ideas and reflected them in their own work. But rather than being of merely historical interest, Hobbes's ideas are still ubiquitous today. One example is the rational concept of the *homo economicus* found in economics and social sciences. Contemporary thinkers such as Steven Pinker and John Gray have studied his work, while novelists like Michel Houellebecq endorse his theory that human beings are driven by fear and paranoia.

With hindsight, it is not hard to explain Hobbes's success − more than anyone else, he has shown what humans are capable of. The starting point of his political philosophy are our passions: appetite, desire, love, aversion, hate, joy and grief. According to Hobbes, these passions are neither divided equally among people, nor are they equally strong in each individual. The large differences between people can have a natural as well as a cultural explanation, as Hobbes points out that our passions are influenced by our physical condition (or, as we would say today, our DNA) as well as our differences in upbringing. While he was sceptical about accounts of witches and supernatural explanations of our behaviour, his books deal extensively with madness, which in the 17th century included hysteria. He defined a hysterical person as someone who has 'stronger, and more vehement passions for anything, than is ordinarily seen in others'.[1] In line with the thinking of his time, Hobbes blamed hysteria on the patient's vital organs, claiming, in a circular argument, that hysteria is caused by the malfunctioning of the organs of the body, which in turn is the result of the severity and duration of hysteria.

For a better understanding of the current thinking about security, we need to take a closer look at the connection Hobbes made between the passions of human beings and their craving for power. In Hobbes, everything is about power. It is not just the strongest of all passions, but the one all other passions derive from, as 'means to obtain some future apparent good'.[2] Hobbes considered the pursuit of wealth and knowledge honourable, because it is a sign of our ability to gain power. He differentiated between natural and instrumental power, defining natural power as exceptional physical or mental endowments such as physical attractiveness and eloquence that allow us to achieve things. Instrumental power, on the other hand, is defined as the abilities we have gained through our natural power or that are given to us by fate, and which we use to acquire more power. Examples of this include having ample financial means, or friends in high places.

In a view that differs considerably from that of thinkers like Spinoza, Hobbes considered the craving for power to be the primary driving force of human behaviour. According to Hobbes, this constant and restless craving for more and more power is humanity's most important driving force − all people share this desire, and it only ends in death. You could sum it up by concluding that human beings can never have enough power; our craving for it results on the one hand from a universal human hope of getting more pleasure out of life, and on the other from a fear of losing the power we already have. Add to this the fact that all people share an equal desire for the same things and a similar hope of achieving their goals, and the picture is complete. Driven by a constant lack and a ceaseless craving for power, everyone is constantly prepared to fight everyone else. To make his deterministic view of human nature even clearer, Hobbes writes:

> And therefore if any two men desire the same thing, which nevertheless they cannot both enjoy, they become enemies; and in the way to their end, (which is principally their own conservation, and sometimes their delectation only) endeavour to destroy or subdue one another.[3]

Kill or be killed

And so it begins. People want more and more power so as to live a decent life, but a world in which everyone is trying to maximise their power is a world full of conflict, ruled by survival of the fittest. Hobbes is clear on this – the pursuit of power in all its variations such as wealth, honour and authority, leads to arguments between citizens, to violence and eventually even to war. He calls this the state of nature, which he presents a hypothetical, fictitious state that has never really existed. In some passages of his work, however, Hobbes refers to the state of nature as a historical fact, such as when he writes about pre-colonial America and the stateless Native Americans living in Virginia and Bermuda. In *De Cive*, he even compares the state of nature to the way people behaved towards each other in the English Civil War.

The notion of the state of nature as a pre-societal life is based on a number of presumptions, one of the most important of which is that there are no political or legal institutions that can prevent violence between citizens. The state of nature is literally a state of 'an-archy' ('without rule'). There are no laws, no police, no army and no judges. Everyone is sovereign. The consequences of this can be seen in the 2013 movie *The Purge*, in which a society allows its citizens to commit any crime they like – even murder – on one night a year. On this so-called crime day, there are no police on duty and hospitals remain closed. The idea behind this is that if people are allowed to do anything they want on one night, they will live together in peace and harmony for the rest of the year.

In the state of nature, the causes of violence fall into roughly three categories: competition, pride and distrust. These passions are constantly causing conflict between people. Competition is of an economic nature: in order to survive, people need certain commodities which often turn out to be scarce, such as food and decent accommodation. A shortage of such things can spark fierce fighting in which people use violence to obtain goods from others or to gain power over them. Pride is a second cause of conflict. According to Hobbes, people are so bent on protecting their reputation that they repay any kind of disdain with violence. The third and last cause is distrust – people harbour a deep mutual distrust of one another, because they know that in principle, others might attack at any moment. Everyone is out for everyone else's blood or possessions. This distrust is continuously fuelled by people always wanting to be one step ahead of one another, until such time that no one else has the power to pose a threat to them anymore.

Because of all these conflicts that come with the natural state, Hobbes calls it a state of war, a 'war of all against all', in which it is either kill or be killed. This does not take large groups of hot-tempered people actually coming to blows; according to Hobbes, it is all about the will to war being generally understood and creating a permanent threat of warfare. This ensures that, even in our society, there is always the possibility of a state of war. Following Gilles Deleuze's line of thinking, you could even argue that the state of war is a diagram of our society – lying dormant, it could break out again at any given moment. On the subject of this special statute on the state of war, which is anchored at the very heart our society, Hobbes argues:

> For war consists not in battle only or the act of fighting; but in a tract of time, wherein the will to contend in battle is sufficiently known; and therefore the notion of time, is to be considered in the nature of war; as it is in the nature of weather. For as the nature of foul weather lies not in the shower or two of rain; but in an inclination thereto of many days together.[4]

The constant fear of others and the threat of a violent death makes people want to leave the state of nature behind them. Without freedom from fear and chaos there can be no work, no shipping industry, no architecture, no engineering, no account of time, no arts, no letters, nor any kind of society, to paraphrase the most frequently quoted passage from *Leviathan*. For this reason, people hope to be able to lead a peaceful and safe life by themselves appointing a higher power who puts an end to the state of complete anarchy. Only an absolute sovereign can keep people's tendency to destroy each other in check and end the fear and violence. In this way, the state of nature is replaced by a nation state, and the only price we have to pay is giving up a significant slice of our freedom.

The monster Leviathan

Hobbes's method of portraying the state of nature is the opposite of utopianism. Rather than sketching a model society like Plato did in his famous work *The Republic*, he describes the horrors of a lawless, unsafe world, and the causes underlying this constant insecurity. Hobbes believed that the only way out of this permanent state of insecurity is appointing a ruler whose most important task is guaranteeing the citizens' safety. To prevent a relapse into the state of nature, the sovereign is given extensive powers, including legislative powers and the monopoly on using force. This means the sovereign is charged with resolving disputes between citizens, levying taxes and punishing lawbreakers, as well as being the warlord who declares war and makes peace.

Hobbes depicts the sovereign as Leviathan from the Old Testament, a Phoenician sea monster that is slain by Yahweh. Besides in the title, Hobbes mentions Leviathan three times in the book, suggesting by the metaphor that the state can become just as strong as this horrifying monster if the people transfer their rights to a sovereign, preferably a single ruler rather than a body of representatives of the people. But while Hobbes uses the sea monster to symbolise the power of a sovereign protecting the world from the fear and violence that reign in the state of nature, the term 'Leviathan' is problematic. Why does Hobbes use this name, which in Christendom symbolises fear and violence, for the sovereign – the very person meant to put an end to the dangerous way of life of the state of nature?

It is worth noting that Leviathan is mentioned six times in the Old Testament: twice in the Psalms, twice in the Book of Isaiah and twice in the Book of Job. In these passages, Leviathan appears in the form of a wide variety of dangerous, monstrous creatures: a snake, a crocodile and a sea serpent. But even if the Bible does not provide an unambiguous image of the Leviathan, its function is less ambiguous. In Job 40, for example, the Leviathan is depicted as a primal force of nature far superior to human capabilities. To illustrate the monster's power, God asks Job the rhetorical question, 'Can you catch Leviathan with your fishing rod? And tie down his tongue with a rope?' (Job 40:24–25). Another monster makes an appearance in the Book of Job. Not a sea serpent this time, but a land monster called Behemoth, a hippopotamus-like beast with a tail like a cedar and enormously powerful abdominal muscles and loins. Just as Leviathan, Behemoth appears in different Old Testament texts as an apocalyptic monster, a creature spat out by Hell itself that does everything in its power to disrupt the lives of humans.

To this day, a fascination for Leviathan has been deeply rooted in our culture. The sea monster has been a popular subject in literature, film and music. In mediaeval times, Leviathan was identified with the devil who oppresses people and leads them into temptation, as in the works of Thomas Aquinas and Jacob van Maerlant, among others. The monster also features in Victor Hugo's famous 1862 book *Les Misérables*, in which the Paris sewer system is described as 'the intestines of Leviathan', and makes regular appearances in popular culture of the 21st century. In the eponymous film by the Russian director Andrey Zvyagintsev (2014), for example, the protagonists Kolya, a labourer living in a fishing village on the Barents Sea with his wife and son, refuses to sell his parental home to the corrupt mayor. When Mayor Sergeyevich employs increasingly aggressive methods to get his hands on the house, resistance seems futile, especially when the powers that be – the police, judiciary and even the church – take his side. In the comic book *Batman Incorporated* published by DC Comics in 2011, the winged superhero takes on an Al-Qa'ida-like organisation called 'Leviathan'. Batman raises an international army of Batmen and Batwomen to win the battle, whose mission is 'to fight ideas with better ideas'.[5]

These references to the monster may seem very different from each other, the depiction of Leviathan as an evil or chaotic power bent on disrupting the existing order is the same. But what does our deep-rooted fascination for the anti-Christian monster tell us about how we currently deal with security? What have monsters got to do with it?

Homo homini lupus

Hobbes describes the human being as a predator who is continually looking for war. This view of humankind flows from his negative anthropology, in which humans are driven by self-preservation and the lust for power. He writes much less, if at all, about such positive passions as hope, love or affection. In a telling line of an autobiographical poem, Hobbes speaks of fear and himself being born together, as twins: 'It was my mother dear / Did bring forth twins at once, both me and fear'. The chapter that Hobbes dedicates to human passions deals mainly with desire, anxiety, fear and hate. Love is barely mentioned. Not only is fear stronger than love, but other people are, by nature, not to be trusted – let alone loved. If Hobbes speaks of love at all, he uses a rather clinical definition of the term and a highly materialistic view of the emotion, which he equates with desire – the only difference being that desire refers to the absence of its object and love to its presence. And, as he remarks dispassionately, love is always accompanied by a certain amount of pleasure. This reduces love to a mere sum of experiences, taking place against a background of a state of nature that is not characterised by love and cooperation but by violence and war; instead of cooperation and solidarity, a win–win situation, the only options here are winning or losing.[6]

Hobbes's deeply cynical view of humans as solitary animals, driven by fear and animosity to take out their anger on each other, is expressed in the metaphor *Homo homini lupus*. This Latin expression that appears in *De Cive* from 1642, means 'A man is a wolf to another man', or put differently, 'Humans are wolves to their fellow humans'. With it, Hobbes distanced himself from the Aristotelian view of human beings as naturally political and social animals. The wolf, by contrast, symbolises the violence latent in humans and the constant threat they pose to others. Hobbes's pessimistic view of humankind was supposedly informed by the times he lived in, and in which he witnessed plague epidemics, civil and religious wars as well as the violence of the Inquisition. Yet the phrase *Homo homini lupus* is not his – it had been used by authors preceding him, including Desiderius Erasmus in *Adagia* (1500), François Rabelais in *Tiers livre* (1546) and Francis Bacon in *De Dignitate et Augmentis Scientiarum* (1623). But most of all, the quote echoes a passage from the comedy *Asinaria* written by the Roman playwright Plautus in the 2nd century BCE. The play is about a father who helps his son get enough money to buy a mistress of his own, so he will not have to share one with other clients anymore. In exchange, the father wants to spend the first night with the woman. The following quote from the comedy is taken from a dialogue between an Athenian donkey merchant and the slave Leonida.

LEONIDA: I could say this now: no one's accused me deservedly yet and there isn't any other man in Athens these days who people believe can be trusted equally well.

DONKEY MERCHANT: Perhaps. Still, you'll never get me to entrust you with this money today because I don't know you. Man is a wolf and not a man toward a man when he doesn't know what he is like.

LEONIDA: Now you're obliging me already.

If we take a closer look at this dialogue in the comedy *Asinaria* and the use it makes of the wolf metaphor, we find that the original expression is not just longer, but also richer in meaning than its counterpart in Hobbes. It seems that Hobbes pared down Plautus's original expression to an aggressive sound bite, so as to bring his point across that we are so distrustful and jealous we lash out at the slightest provocation. In the Latin original of *Asinaria*, Plautus writes, '*Lupus est homo homini, non homo, quom qualis sit non novit*', which roughly translates as, 'When he does not know him, a man is no man to his fellow men, but a wolf.' It is striking that the original text emphasises the quality of the relationship between people, making this relationship, the knowledge people have of one another, crucial to human interaction. You can only know something about another person once you have made contact, when you open yourself to others and get to know one another. This may not always be an agreeable experience – interacting with others can bring unpleasant things to light – but you make a connection, which according to Plautus is the most important thing. This does not happen when one person immediately bashes another's brains in.

Hobbes's raw realism has not lost any of its explanatory power. His version of the expression *Homo homini lupus* has become one of the cornerstones of the way we view humans. Arthur Schopenhauer quotes Hobbes with palpable relish in his 1818 book *Die Welt als Wille und Vorstellung*, in which he writes, 'The chief source of the most serious evils afflicting man is man himself; *homo homini lupus.*'[7] Sigmund Freud also adopts Hobbes's characterisation of humans as egotistical and aggressive creatures. In *Das Unbehagen in der Kultur* from 1930, he argues:

Men are not gentle creatures, who want to be loved, who at the most can defend themselves if they are attacked; they are, on the contrary, creatures among whose instinctual endowments is to be reckoned a powerful share of aggressiveness. [...] Homo homini lupus. Who in the face of all his experience of life and of history, will have the courage to dispute this assertion?[8]

More recent proof of Hobbes's ideas still being very much alive can be found in the work of conservative criminologists, such as Thomas Hirschi and James Q. Wilson, who depart from the Hobbesian assumption that the individual is dangerous and potentially evil and that crime requires a rigorous response by the police and criminal justice system. It can also be found in the writings of the British biologist Richard Dawkins. In the last paragraph of his 1976 book on the evolutionary importance of genes, *The Selfish Gene*, he writes that evolution is purely driven by the reproduction of the self-serving gene. According to Dawkins, the challenge is to learn to become generous and altruistic, or else remain egotists. Slavoj Žižek, whose work also remains in the shadow of Hobbes, believes that humans are malicious and egotistic by nature – anything positive we do is chiefly designed to make us feel good.

All the animals come out at night

In the last decade, Thomas Hobbes's view of human nature has become more relevant than ever. In a period in which terrorist attacks appear to be more violent and frequent than they had been for a long time, the wolf rears its vile head again. An increasing number of suicide bombers appear to be acting on their own account, without the help or schooling of a terrorist organisation. Such terrorists are called lone wolves, because they operate and attack on their own like a solitary wolf. The term 'lone wolf' has become so popularised in recent years that it now covers a wide variety of terrorist. If we take a closer look at the term, we see that it has dissolved in a variety of different categories and simplistic generalisations. Everything has been lumped together under it, from solitary Jihadists to far right terrorists. A classic example of the lone wolf is Volkert van der Graaf, the murderer of the Dutch politician Pim Fortuyn, who did not belong to, or receive instructions from, any group or terrorist network with a clear organisation and chain of command.

Despite their great diversity however, lone wolves have in common that they feel superior to everyone who does not share their point of view, and that they regard themselves as heroes or soldiers. The Kouachi brothers, for example, carried out their 2015 attack on the French Charlie Hebdo magazine in military uniforms, and the Norwegian Anders Breivik wore a police uniform during his twin attacks in Norway in 2011, killing 77 people. The favoured target of lone wolves is someone who symbolises the government they despise, particularly soldiers and police officers. But while they may look like twisted loners at first sight, lone wolves do not operate in a social vacuum. They post detailed messages on Instagram and reactions in the comments sections of YouTube videos by Islamic State, in which young people are encouraged to carry out terrorist attacks. They also claim to be acting for a greater purpose which they share with others. Many attacks are triggered by strong feelings of outrage about issues that are currently present in society, such as civil rights, immigration and Islam. The attackers frequently leave messages for their family and friends, or drop hints on the internet about their planned attack.

The lone wolf as a product of Western culture is portrayed most aptly in the 1976 movie *Taxi Driver*, by Martin Scorsese. There are examples of the Hobbesian view of humans as aggressive and egotistic predators in almost all of Scorsese's films – ranging from the explosive gangsters in *Goodfellas* (1990) and *Casino* (1995) to the overstrung boxer Jake LaMotta in *Raging Bull* (1980), and from the intensely vindictive psychopath Max Cady in *Cape Fear* (1991) to the aggressive amoral stockbroker Jordan Belfort in *The Wolf of Wall Street* (2013). But of all his films, it is most pronounced in *Taxi Driver*, in which Robert de Niro plays the frustrated, 26-year-old war veteran Travis Bickle, who is planning to carry out an attack on the presidential candidate Charles Palantine during one of his campaign speeches. The protagonist goes through life as an outsider, wrapped in a cocoon of loneliness – in an interview on the theme of the film, Scorsese emphasises that Bickle is unable to commit to a relationship. He is a lone wolf cruising aimlessly around the depraved neighbourhoods of New York, a world very similar to Hobbes's state of nature, in which everything is in decay and the law of the jungle rules. In one of the most famous scenes of the film, Travis Bickle reads from his diary: 'All the animals come out at night – whores, dopers, junkies, sick, venal. Someday a real rain will come and wash all this scum off the streets.'

The number of lone wolves has risen sharply in recent years. Between 1940 and 2000, 39 lone wolves were active, but this number had risen to over 70 in the period between 2000 and 2018. Nevertheless, the metaphor of the lone wolf also raises questions. Does the Hobbesian image of the wolf as a solitary predator really give us a better understanding of human beings? And how has this image influenced security hysteria?

Wolf hysteria

The wolf has had a bad reputation since time immemorial – all of our hysteria seems packed together in the image of the 'big bad wolf'. Old European folk tales and fairy tales are full of warnings about this animal, which was considered Satan in disguise, or his projection in humans. Stories ranging from Little Red Riding Hood to Disney's Zeke Wolf, and from Dracula to the Wolf and the Seven Young Goats, all depict the wolf as an aggressive and bloodthirsty beast that kills more animals than it eats. Even today, wolf sightings create a stir and heightened alertness. Far right parties such as the German Alternative für Deutschland portray the wolf as an 'immigrant' that poses a threat to children and family life but is protected by the 'elites'. Committees are formed, and in several countries national contingency plans are in place so as to be ready if and when the wolf arrives. According to such guidelines, people should 'speak loudly and gesticulate' if a wolf gets too close.

All things considered, it is strange that the wolf has such a bad reputation – for of all wild animals, it is closest to humans. In their fascinating 2017 book *The First Domestication*, Raymond Pierotti and Brandy Fogg demonstrate in countless examples that humans and wolves had been inseparable companions for a long period of time. Nor was this a one-sided relationship in which the wolves dominated; on the contrary, early humans learned a great deal from wolves. Pierotti and Fogg call this the 'lupification of human behaviour'. The Blackfoot People (NiiTsitapiiksi) for example, used to live closely with wolves in parts of Western Canada and what is now the US State of Montana. The wolves joined them hunting bison, and the Native Americans shared their food with them. Whenever a wolf approached a hunting party, the Native Americans sang, 'No, I will not give you my body to eat, but I will give you the body of someone else, if you will join us.'

The wolf is also the first animal to be domesticated by humans, long before we did the same with cattle, sheep, goats and pigs. A docile lapdog is in fact nothing else but a watered-down version of a wolf. But the most important point is that unlike Travis Bickle in *Taxi Driver*, the wolf is not a loner – just like humans, it is a social animal that is a member of a family and works together closely with others in packs. An average pack of about ten animals consists of parents and their young, often from different years. In areas like Alaska where prey is plentiful, the number of wolves in a pack can reach between 20 and 30 animals. It goes without saying that they sometimes fight among themselves and can be cruel to one another, but outside of a pack, a wolf has very little chance of survival. When a young adult wolf leaves its family, it goes in search of a wolf of the opposite sex in order to settle in an area outside of its parental territory. Young wolves sometimes leave the pack to go hunting on their own but they usually return very soon; wolves can only hunt in groups in which each animal has its own tasks to perform. A pack is organised according to a strict hierarchy led by an alpha male and female, and each animal in it has its own role and responsibility. It also gives meaning to the wolf's existence; just like human families, a pack is a social unit that provides the wolves with safety and security. A pack that stays together is safest for all its members.

The Dutch primatologist and ethologist Frans De Waal has also been a vocal critic of Hobbes's view of humans as wolves. In *The Age of Empathy*, published in 2009, he rejects Hobbes's theory that we are hard-wired for aggression and violence. Basing himself on his biological fieldwork, De Waal argues that we descend from a long line of primates that lived in groups and were heavily dependent on one another. Behavioural traits such as loving and caring for each other can be found in two types of anthropoid apes that are genetically almost identical to us; chimpanzees and bonobos. Anyone studying the social behaviour of these animals must come to the conclusion that it is entirely normal for animals to work together, and that the positive passions of humans are deeply rooted in evolutionary processes. De Waal considers reconciliation, which is a major human behavioural trait and one of the main themes of his work, as our shared heritage with apes, and believes it has the function of strengthening group cohesion. Humans may be violent and aggressive, but we are also social and empathic by nature. In *The Bridge to Humanity* from 2006, Walter Goldschmidt calls this 'affect hunger', the urge to get expressions of affection from others. This need for connection is just a strong as the need for a full stomach. I will expand on this subject in the next chapter.

If it bleeds, we can kill it

Our fascination with the monster Leviathan shows how much we are still enthralled by magical and mystical creatures – however much such authors as Max Weber (disenchantment), Eduard Jan Dijksterhuis (mechanisation) and Norbert Elias (civilising) would like to convince us of the opposite. Without wishing to exaggerate the role of cinema, film is undoubtedly the most potent mirror of all that is monstrous in our culture. Personifying our deepest fears, monsters feed our society's hysteria about the unknown and the obscure. A quick search reveals countless examples of movies about our reasonable and unreasonable fears of everything monstrous. In fact, we find most of our fears reflected in movies – the fear of terrorists, viruses, immigrants, clowns – are all up there on the big screen.

Arguably, the best movies tell you something about the spirit of the times in which they come out. In the 1950s, for example, the memory of the horrors of the Second World War were still so fresh that this provided the base material for many films about totalitarian regimes and cruel dictators. A famous example of this is the 1956 adaptation of George Orwell's novel *1984*, as is *Invasion of the Body Snatchers*, another film about communism from the same year, and François Truffaut's *Fahrenheit 451* from 1966, starring Oskar Werner and Julie Christie. Three excellently acted movies that explore censorship and other intrusive forms of control that governments exert on their citizens, and examine the existence of all kinds of oppression and domination by asking questions on who decides on the implementation of new technology, and what happens to our freedom when privacy no longer exists.

Times change, and movies change along with them. In the 1970s, the focus of cinema shifted to the survival of our planet. This was prompted by the famous 1972 report *The Limits of Growth* that was drawn up by the Club of Rome, a think tank of scientists and industrialists. The Club used computer models to make predictions for the period until the year 2100, based on five parameters – the world economy, pollution, food production, population growth and use of natural resources – and predicted that our major resources would be depleted within a few decades. Nine million copies of the report were sold worldwide – 300,000 in the Netherlands alone within mere months – while the headline of the Dutch newspaper *NRC Handelsblad* read, 'World Threatened by Disaster'. The widespread social anxiety about the future of the planet was reflected on the big screen in such environmentally aware films as *Z.P.G.* (1972), *Silent Running* (1972), *Soylent Green* (1973) and *Logan's Run* (1976), which explore the consequences of overpopulation and extreme pollution, and the possibility of a toxic future.

The 1980s saw an increase of public concern in the Western world about the steeply rising crime rate and the spread of violence in big cities. In the early 1980s, there was a sharp rise in violent crime in the United Kingdom and the United States, and New York even became known as the crime capital of the world. The enormous social impact of this was reflected in movies which show that the law and order in our society is not in fact as stable as people think; chaos and anarchy are lying in wait because of alien elements threatening our quiet existence. This has rarely been depicted with such urgency as in the 1979 film *Alien*, in which the cargo spaceship *Nostromo* returns to Earth with a deadly and invisible alien being on board. A ground-breaking masterpiece that blends science fiction with industrial Gothic and body horror, the movie is about the colonisation of Earth by an alien being which, in its microscopic form, embeds itself in the human body. It is no coincidence that the name of the cargo ship *Nostromo* refers to Joseph Conrad's eponymous novel from 1904, in which the author depicts the capitalist violence of high finance as a form of continued colonisation. While the film shows only glimpses of the alien, director Ridley Scott asserts that 'its only point is terror and more terror'. It draws on the worst nightmare imaginable to humans: an invisible evil whose blood is corrosive acid, which spreads death and destructions, feels no guilt and has no ethics.

In *The Thing* by director John Carpenter, released three years later in 1982, a group of scientists excavate a strange, 100,000 year-old creature on Antarctica. Once it has thawed, they watch in horror as the creature begins to mutate into all kinds of shapes, including those of the scientists themselves, which leads to the existential question of who is the human and who the alien. In one of the best scenes in cinema, the scientists run a blood test to find out which one of them is the alien: 'I dunno what the hell's in there, but it's weird and pissed off, whatever it is.' In a later interview, Carpenter called *The Thing* the first part of his 'apocalypse trilogy', of which *Prince of Darkness* (1987) is the second part and *In the Mouth of Madness* (1995) the final one. In 1987, *Predator* hit the cinemas, starring the muscle-bound bodybuilder Arnold Schwarzenegger. Schwarzenegger was never better than in the role of Alan Schaefer, also known as 'Dutch', the leader of a military commando unit. What begins as a typical war movie set in the sweltering jungle of Latin America in which a rescue operation is launched to find the crew of a lost helicopter, turns into a compelling struggle against an intelligent, reptilian alien creature with dreadlocks that remains invisible for most of the film. This predator can detect heat, hides in the jungle and hunts down people for sport. The pivotal phrase of the movie is, 'If it bleeds, we can kill it.'

Film clichés are rarely in line with reality, but there is a remarkable kernel of truth in *Alien, The Thing* and *Predator*. While they may be wildly different movies, the subject of all three of them is a threat coming from outside that changes the world as we know it radically, in the form of an alien or some other dangerous monster that has no clear motivation and is unencumbered by morals. A recurrent theme in these movies is the fear of the strange and the unknown, and the emphasis on the fact that you cannot tell who is actually dangerous. Nobody knows where the danger comes from, the characters are threatened from all sides. It is a type of danger that functions like a virus – when anyone could be infected, everyone could be dangerous.

This list of movies can easily be expanded, but it might be more useful to point out that these are no isolated examples. Images that evoke fear of the strange and the unknown have an enormous impact on the vitality of society and citizens, and have been closely related with the hysterical tenor of Western society – especially in the 1980s, when civilisations and societal values were put on the line by the continually rising crime rate.

Harry Potter language

For some time, monsters have not been confined to the realm of children's stories, but have also served a purpose for the adult imagination. Our relationship with monsters is often a lot less rational than we would have ourselves believe. Everyone remembers the Margaret Thatcher and Ronald Reagan era, characterised by the swing to the right of 1980s politics. The thinking of these two politicians was characterised by a remarkable synthesis between apparently opposing beliefs. According to Thatcher and Reagan, the main problem was that government had become too powerful. They firmly believed in a free market, and projected the neoliberal principles of a market economy onto the general art of leading their countries, which led to the sell-off of state-owned companies and the privatisation of such public services as the post office and gas and water suppliers. At the same time, however, both Thatcher and Reagan were pushing the neoconservative story that they would save their country from the complete ruin it was threatened by from foreign dangers. In a 1978 TV interview, Thatcher described the fears about immigration by implying that the UK 'might be rather swamped by people of a different culture'. The two leaders' recipe for achieving their goals was an almost Eastern European dirigisme: 'Less tax and more law and order.'[9]

While *Alien, The Thing* and *Predator* were showing in cinemas, Thatcher and Reagan peppered their speeches with references to monsters and demons meant to depict lawbreakers. Reagan consistently portrayed criminals as predators or aliens, as for example in a talk he gave in New Orleans in 1981 in which he described a young lawbreaker as follows: 'A stark, staring face – a face that belongs to a frightening reality of our time: the face of the human predator.' In countless public appearances, Reagan, who became president after a successful career in Hollywood, evoked the image of higher, sinister powers on the brink of disrupting the order that had been so painstakingly created by our forefathers. In a speech to the United Nations on 21 September 1987, he told the audience:

> In our obsession with antagonisms of the moment, we often forget how much unites all the members of humanity. Perhaps we need some outside,

universal threat to make us recognize this common bond. I occasionally think how quickly our differences worldwide would vanish if we were facing an alien threat from outside this world. And yet, I ask you, is not an alien force already among us?[10]

A search through the White House archives shows that in his eight years as president of the United States, Reagan and his wife Nancy watched almost 400 films. The couple shared a preference for the work of Steven Spielberg, director of such movies as *ET*, in which an alien creature lands on Earth and is pursued by American secret services. There is no telling how much Reagan's viewing habits influenced his political decisions, but it is certain that in his presidency, the line between fact and fiction often became blurred. Reagan used film language in countless public appearances to play on his audience's basic instincts and insecurities, for instance while speaking of the United States' precarious situation in the early 1980s. In a 1981 speech to the International Association of Chiefs of Police, Reagan warned of an invisible evil about to invade American society: 'For all our science and sophistication, for all our justified pride in intellectual accomplishment, we should never forget: the jungle is always there, waiting to take us over'. Reagan's reference to the jungle was not innocently made – nor was it a mere figure of speech. As we know from Karl Marx, naming a thing increases its value, creating something that was not there before.[11] The 'jungle' describes more than just a tropical rainforest; rather, it refers to a primordial area dominated by predators that exudes an eerie energy – the concrete jungle of the big city. Reagan's jungle is the ultimate horror movie in which something outside of ourselves, which does not have our best interests at heart, takes over society.

Just like the philosophical language of Hobbes, Reagan's film language had an important social function. The image he sketched of the Hobbesian jungle populated by predatory wild animals is also one of hope, suggesting that when it comes down to it, we have a government to save us from the scary monsters. This is why Reagan considered the police as 'the thin blue line that holds back a jungle which threatens to reclaim this clearing we call civilization'. He constantly used terms that referred to war tactics, such as 'battlefield', 'military intelligence', 'the deployment of the armed forces', 'battle' and 'crusade'.[12] Combined with his knowing glance, dramatic timing and facial expressions, the tone of the film was set – featuring in the lead role a strong and sovereign nation state with strict security policies in place to deal with everyone and everything that harboured bad intentions. This also goes some way to explaining the US's punitive agenda of increasingly harsh sentencing, strict prison regimes (boot camps) and frequent capital punishment. In the struggle against such forces as chaos and ignorance, those would later be complemented by curfews and 'naming & shaming' practices, such as publicising the names and addressed of paedophiles who have served their sentences.

It would be a mistake, however, to think that Reagan's sinister film language was a typically American phenomenon, a rhetorical mood-setting device that could only exist in the country of Hollywood and Broadway. Where fighting crime and disorder is concerned, police forces in other Western countries also have a knack for speaking of good and evil in Harry Potter language. As an example, the Dutch police wrote in the *Politie in ontwikkeling* (Police In Transition) report that the aim of the police force is to 'de-anonymise, identify and call a halt to evil'.[13] One unfortunate result of this use of language, which differentiates between just two kinds of people in the world and which imagines evil as an autonomous and anonymous force, is that it increases the government's power and decreases legal protection of citizens. You could also say that when someone is framed as the 'enemy', it comes as no surprise that they are treated as such.

How people become monsters

Fear of monsters is an important ingredient of hysteria. When the monsters we are confronted with have human faces, this fear can quickly turn into mass hysteria. Until well into the 19th century, the definition of a monster was a creature with serious physical abnormalities. It was considered a phenomenon that defied the laws of nature and did not have a human appearance. Today, however, anyone who deviates from the norm is a little bit monstrous. By this I mean abnormal individuals who have internalised their monstrousness, making them visually unrecognisable as monsters.[14] Movies like *Alien* and *The Thing* show us that they can come in two different varieties. The one that appeals to the imagination the most, is the monster taking over one specific individual, crushing this person's soul as it were and abruptly turning them evil and aggressive. If anyone is liable to be presented as this type of monster today, it is the man who cannot keep his hands off young children. This 'filthy paedo', as he is known today, is viewed as an unscrupulous two-legged sexual monster that needs to be banned from society once and for all. The other type of monster takes possession of an entire group of people and manifests itself in gradually changing security policies. Such policies are based on vague nightmare visions and stereotypes relating to people's ethnicity, ranging from Moroccan youth to radicalised Muslims. The over-representation of these groups in certain forms of crime is alternately explained by 'Moroccan culture' and 'Islam',[15] a practice that the Canadian philosopher Ian Hacking has called 'making up people'.[16]

While fear of monsters is a multifaceted and complex phenomenon, it does follow a discernible logic. It can make emotions run so high that we no longer dare to face these monsters out of fear that things will get even worse, resulting in the hysterical rhetoric becoming reality and leading to far-reaching measures that are out of all proportion to the seriousness of the danger. A severe penalty like exile is a good example of this. Banishing undesirables from the community has had a long history – ever since antiquity, all kinds of people have been physically removed from villages, cities or countries. These people were taken past the city's boundary stone (also called *banpaal*, ban post, in Dutch) and forbidden to ever cross the boundaries of the city again. The meaning of the word 'ban' is reflected in 'bandit', which denotes a villain, gangster or criminal, and literally means 'banished thief'. The word derives from the Italian, where highwaymen were known as bandits. In ancient texts, the banished criminal is deemed equivalent to a wolf-man (wargus) or werewolf, a half human, half animal hiding in between urban and rural areas, where the difference between humans and animals is blurred.[17]

The methods we use today to remove those from society who make us feel uneasy are just as physical as in the past – examples include the removal of loitering teens, beggars, the homeless, addicts, prostitutes, shoplifters and 'confused individuals' from public spaces. At this point we might well ask ourselves if the truly monstrous presence is not 'the creature' itself but the political system responsible for its creation which never improves the well-being of those who are worst-off. Under the pretext of vague, wide-ranging notions of public safety such as a 'clean, intact and safe' environment, these people are treated like lepers, the idea being that such factors as 'clean' and 'intact' are inextricably linked with the level of safety in a neighbourhood or area. A poorly maintained neighbourhood in physical disarray, full of litter, vacant houses and graffiti, is thought to make the inhabitants believe they live in an unmanaged and unmanageable part of the city, and to lead to a steep rise in crime and disorder. James Wilson and George Kelling's broken windows theory that is based on this premise – the best-known American export product in the field of security – asserts that physical and social disorder are conducive to crime. 'If a window in a building is broken', Wilson and Kelling wrote in *The Atlantic Monthly* in 1982, 'and is left unrepaired, all the rest of the windows will soon be broken.' Shortly afterwards drugs will change hands, prostitutes will solicit, and cars will be stripped. This makes it essential that streets and neighbourhood are kept clean and intact. Trash attracts trash.

British anthropologist Mary Douglas would argue that the broken windows theory says everything about the way in which we treat things we consider 'dirty'. The main idea of her 1966 book *Purity and Danger* is that all peoples know the twin terms 'dirty' and 'clean', but that their definitions vary widely. Nothing is dirty or filthy in itself. What is considered clean in one place can be dirty in the next; there is no such thing as 'absolute dirt'. 'Dirt' depends on the context, it is 'a matter out of place'. Douglas shows that the difference between 'dirty' and 'clean' has everything to do with the way in which we bring order to our lives. Our desire for purity and our need to remove dirt does not stem from a fear of disease, as anthropologists believed for a long time, but is linked with a deeper need to mark our territory. In this regard, Douglas writes, the meaning of the term 'dirt' is instrumental as well as expressive. Its instrumental meaning lies in the fact that a collective fear of and aversion to dirt binds people together and instils a degree of respect in them for social standards.

Additionally, statements about what is 'dirty' and what is 'clean' are among the most powerful means of drawing the line between good and evil, normal and abnormal, us and them.

We want the experience we have in our public spaces to be 'clean, intact and safe', which is also increasingly what policy-makers aim at. A quick look around reveals public spaces full of concrete flower pots acting as roadblocks, digital security gates, 'sadistic street furniture' meant to deter people from lying down on it, private security guards, barriers, surveillance cameras and a host of other monitoring and detection devices. Moreover, the police have the power to stop and search without suspicion, and area bans for shoplifters and troublemakers are seen as a panacea for crime.[18] Thanks to an obsession with cleanliness in our society, which can be traced back to so-called primitive cultures and religions and a fear of anything that deviates from prevailing norms, such area bans are gradually creeping up the agenda. In the 21st century, a 'clean' environment is one without graffiti, smashed windows, broken street furniture, burst bin bags or litter. But 'clean' also means that more and more areas are purged of people that do not belong there, or who look intimidating or disorderly; 'social trash', in other words. Such monsters must be removed as quickly as possible, before they disrupt our carefully ordered lives. Good riddance to bad rubbish.

Conclusion

As the work of Immanuel Kant, John Stuart Mill and John Rawls shows, the Enlightenment provided the image of humans as autonomous beings driven by logic and reason who do not let themselves be carried away by their feelings and passions. But the era also laid the foundation of the view that humans are evil and dangerous by nature, which still informs the way we treat criminals and deal with their irrationality, aggression, violence and immoral behaviour. The criminal is no longer a fellow human being who has taken a wrong turn in life, but a dangerous animal that must be banished from society. In his *Second Treatise of Civil Government*, the British early Enlightenment philosopher John Locke compares the criminal to 'a lion or a tiger, one of those wild savage beasts, with whom men can have no society nor security'.[19] All of this goes back to Hobbes's classic theory of the natural condition of human beings as one of constant aggression towards one another, which can only be rectified by appointing a higher power: Leviathan. This may all sound very rational, but it seems to me that when envisaging Leviathan, Hobbes believed above all that the violence of humans could only be countered by pitting their animal side against themselves – in the form of a more brutal, cruel and stronger monster than the wolf. Leviathan has replaced the wolf – an Überwolf that surpasses all other wolves.

Many claim that the world is a less magical place than it used to be, but this is often not the case. On the contrary, the above shows that governments still needs a fantasy world full of horrible monsters to justify their existence, and that the ostentatiously rational world of politics and law enforcement is actually based on the magical world of myths and monsters. It is important to note that rather than an escape from reality, these monsters are a way of clarifying the abnormal. You could even say that monsters shape our identity by showing us who we do not want to be. One of the monsters that appeal to our imagination the most is the criminal, who, by breaking the social contract, reverts to the bloody battlefield of the state of nature in which security is not the opposite of fear and enmity, but their result.[20] With hindsight, you could argue that this misconception has led us to view security as the absence of fear and enmity – a scant definition if ever there was one. And it is precisely that misconception which has led to the current, completely hysterical situation in which security policies are based on firm action and severe punishment and accompanied by unadulterated, tough military language levelled against everything that deviates from the norms.

If security is an extension of war with other means, the question inevitably arises under what conditions this war will be allowed to end. When will there be an end to all of this prohibiting and combating? Who will sign the peace treaty that ends security hysteria? No one seems to know, and I believe this is because no such conditions can be defined. There is no way of telling exactly when we are completely safe, nor can there be a society without crime. Besides, we find it impossible to imagine an alternative to a society that revolves around war; even peace is defined as the absence of war, a definition which is dictated by militant thinking. But an alternative narrative is nevertheless needed, as it is the only thing that can emancipate us from thinking in terms of warfare, and consequently of the hysteria that has ensconced itself in our notions of security.

Notes

1 Hobbes (2003, p. 60).
2 Hobbes (2003, p. 70).
3 Hobbes (2003, p. 100).
4 Hobbes (2003, p. 101).
5 In his book *De Leviathan toen en nu*, Bob Becking (2015) brilliantly depicts Leviathan's comeback in popular culture.
6 Hobbes did not accept that the state had a relation of 'care' towards those whose lives it administered, but rather a relation of justice, writes Frédéric Gros in *The Security Principle* (Gros 2019, p. 143).
7 Schopenhauer (1844, p. 575).
8 Freud (2006e, p. 502).
9 At the beginning of the 1980s, Operation Swamp 81, a new police stop-and-search policy named after Margaret Thatcher's comments, was deployed to reduce street crime in London. In the first six days of the operation, 943 people – the vast majority of them black male youths – were stopped by plain-clothes officers (Bowling, Parmar & Phillips 2003).
10 Ronald Reagan, 'Address to the 42d Session of the United Nations General Assembly in New York', 21 September 1987, retrieved from www.reaganlibrary.gov/archives/sp eech/address-42d-session-united-nations-general-assembly-new-york-new-york

11 Three years after the release of the 1983 movie *WarGames*, the US Congress implemented the Computer Fraud and Abuse Act, which made hacking punishable by law. In the film, Matthew Broderick plays a whizz-kid who understands computers better than his schoolwork and is addicted to video games. To get new games, he hacks random companies, until one day he accidentally hacks into the mainframe computer of the US Army and almost unleashes a Third World War.

12 Stuart (2011, p. 9). American writer Susan Sontag writes in *Illness as Metaphor* about the ways in which military metaphors such as 'war', waged on diseases ranging from cancer to AIDS, are used to displace complex situations into metaphors of grim battles that must be won at all costs. According to Sontag, 'the transformation of war-making into an occasion for mass ideological mobilization has made the notion of war useful as a metaphor for all sorts of ameliorative campaigns whose goals are cast as the defeat of an "enemy"' (Sontag 1990, pp. 98–99).

13 Netherlands Police Institute (2005, p. 90).

14 Other famous examples of outsiders include René Girard's 'scapegoat' (Girard 1988) and Zygmunt Bauman's 'stranger'. In his book *Modernity and Ambivalence*, Bauman writes about strangers: 'These [strangers, MS] are the true hybrids, the monsters – not just unclassified, but unclassifiable. [...] They must be tabooed, disarmed, suppressed, exiled physically or mentally – or the world may perish' (Bauman 1991, pp. 58–59). To an even greater extent than the scapegoat and the stranger, however, the monster is a legal matter, as the law typifies certain people and behaviours as abnormal.

15 It goes without saying that this is a spurious representation. Among other things, certain risk factors for crime, including dropping out of school and unemployment, are more common in certain ethnic groups, but it does not follow that the perpetrators engage in criminal behaviour *because* of their ethnic background.

16 Hacking (1986).

17 The Italian philosopher Giorgio Agamben makes a connection between the criminal and the werewolf, but in a very different way than Hobbes. Agamben believes the werewolf represents a bigger picture, and that the transformation from human to werewolf corresponds with a state of emergency in which the punishment of excommunication links the sovereign to bare life. In *Homo sacer*, Agamben (1998) points out that the criminal can be banished from society by the sovereign, who is the only one with the power of excommunication. The idea of banishment originated in old Germanic law, which made the connection between the outlaw (*Friedlose*) and the banishment the criminal faced.

18 Schuilenburg (2015a).

19 Locke (2015, p. 36).

20 Carney & Dadusc (2014); Neocleous (2019).

Chapter 4

Will the real human being please stand up?

Introduction

In the previous chapter we saw that the influence of Thomas Hobbes has led to a strong tendency to explain human existence in terms of negative behavioural traits. Fear and mistrust are buried deep in our DNA and set the tone for our lives. These negative emotions feed on the human tendency to try to outwit one another. The basic theme of human behaviour according to this view is self-interest. To Hobbes humans are therefore nothing more than *homo egocentricus*, a bestial animal that is first and foremost bad and selfish, and that aggressively strives for self-preservation and fulfilment of its own needs. In fact you might sum up Hobbes as saying that our entire existence is dominated by the 'will to survive'. We find similar ideas reading Adam Smith (humans are led by self-interest), Friedrich Nietzsche (will to power) and Sigmund Freud (humans are innately aggressive).

Hobbes's view of humans continues to cast its shadow on our society. The hysterical dimension is apparent in the way in which we structure society to fit a view of humanity that emphasises evil and requires the government to keep citizens under control, out of fear of civil war. In this view, which puts an emphasis on punishment and substantial exaggeration, security is synonymous with combating insecurity. The consequence of all this is that security policies are easily narrowed down to a question of law enforcement and harsh measures. Add to that citizens' hypersensitivity to the insecurity that remains – 'My country is on fire!' – and you end up with a hysterical view that something must be done or it will be 'the end of civilisation' and 'we'll be thrown to the wolves'.

Plenty of philosophers and scientists criticise the Hobbesian view of humans as bestial animals. While Hobbes peppered us with gunpowder when he declared his pitch-black view of humans, Jean-Jacques Rousseau applied balm when he stated that humans were good by nature – according to his view, it was society that corrupted humans. His contemporary, David Hume, also expressed criticism of Hobbes, arguing that there are elements of the wolf and the snake in humans, but that we also harbour the dove in our hearts. But the most significant criticism comes from the Dutch primatologist and ethologist

Frans De Waal. His work puts considerable pressure on the assumptions behind Hobbes's idea and those of his successors, as he argues that communal living does not arise from a rational social contract. Communal life in fact forms the natural foundation of human existence. In this respect, De Waal reminds us that a society is not based on mutual advantage but rather on organic connections, among which positive behavioural traits such as empathy, friendship, care for others and spontaneous aid are important dimensions of social bonding. In this respect, De Waal reaches back to Aristotle's communitarian vision, stating that humans are by nature socially and politically communal animals – although humans in the Greek *polis* were narrowly defined as men of a certain level of wealth.

Just how brutal and aggressive are humans by nature? Is it possible that Hobbes's gloomy view of humanity and the associated security hysteria are unfounded? Or, to take a phrase from rapper Eminem, 'Will the real human being please stand up?'

Community spirit

Frans De Waal has a talent for picking the right subject at the right time, as well as finding the right way to present it. He's not just an influential scientist; according to *Time Magazine* he is one of the hundred most influential people in the world. He also reaches a broad audience with his intriguing stories about primate behaviour via TV, columns and accessibly written books such as *The Ape and the Sushi Master* (2001) and *The Bonobo and the Atheist* (2013). The message of his work is that we are mistaken in thinking there is a big distance between humans and animals. Although humans have tried for centuries to set themselves apart by characterising themselves as 'political animals' (Aristotle) or as 'the animal whose nature has not yet been fixed' (Nietzsche), De Waal is convinced that animal and human behaviour are in fact very similar. Based on many years observing aggression and reconciliation among groups of apes, he has coined terms such as the 'inner ape' and 'anthropodenial' (denying human traits in animals).

His work does away with the illustrious 'veneer theory', which has long been the dominant view on human nature. Veneer theory holds that deep down, humans are not moral creatures who distinguish good and evil; instead they are selfish and hostile. In line with Hobbes's view of humans, our morality according to this theory is a thin veneer over an amoral core, barely concealing our true nature. Nowhere is this so magnificently represented as in the film *Apocalypse Now*, Francis Ford Coppola's 1979 masterpiece, with the character of the American Colonel Kurtz, played by Marlon Brando. During the Vietnam War, Kurtz goes completely off the rails as his animal instincts take control. The wafer-thin veneer of civilisation vanishes deep in the Cambodian hinterlands, like snow melting in the sun. In an iconic scene, Kurtz talks to Captain Benjamin Willard, who has been tasked with eliminating him, and explains to him in Hobbesian fashion the concept of 'horror': 'Horror has a face, and you must make a friend of horror. Horror and moral terror are your friends. If they are not, then they are enemies to be feared.'

Veneer theory has points in common with the Christian concept of original sin, but is mainly known through the work of the Victorian biologist Thomas Henry Huxley, one of the most fervent defenders of Darwin's theory of evolution. His unflinching defence of Darwin's theory in lectures and debates earned him the nickname 'Darwin's bulldog'. Huxley states that ethics are not a product of evolution and that morality must be kept separate from evolutionary theory. When opponents – unable to imagine the evolutionary advantages of collaboration and altruism – pointed out to him that he was contradicting himself in saying so, he apologised for his lack of logic and famously insisted that this is simply the way things are. Huxley summed up human ethics as a triumph over the dark forces in nature, which continually threaten to drag us into the depths. In doing so he made a comparison with a gardener toiling to maintain his garden and prevent it from becoming wild and overgrown. De Waal refers to this as 'Calvinist sociobiology': only with very hard work will we have any chance of amounting to anything.

In his 2006 book *Primates and Philosophers*, De Waal argues that there are fundamental problems with veneer theory, as this view of morality denies the social aspect of our species. According to De Waal, we have never been atomic individuals lacking community spirit. Group living forms the natural basis of human existence – in fact, De Waal writes, we have always been 'social to the core' even in the natural state of our distant forebears.[1] We have an innate need to collaborate and take responsibility for one another. For instance, our ancestors lived together in small groups, tribal communities with a communal language and religion, in which everything revolved around matters such as loyalty, care and protection. For the people in these groups, communal living was not an option but a survival strategy. Cooperation and proximity were necessary in order to survive and offered us protection against predators. Without collaboration you were condemned to death.

Veneer theory also runs into difficulties explaining how we evolved from amoral animals into moral creatures. Morality did not drop out of the sky; we did not turn social overnight. De Waal therefore does not endorse Hobbes's social contract theory, which explains society as the result of rational agreements our ancestors made in their natural state which continue to form the basis of social living now, and security as an answer to the fear and violence of the natural state. As we saw in the previous chapter, this means in a philosophical sense that security is not in opposition to fear and enmity, but that it is the direct effect of them, because self-interest drives us to hand over our freedom to a higher power – Leviathan – which in turn offers us protection. But according to De Waal the idea that our ancestors gave up their freedom in exchange for security is an erroneous origin myth. Security is not the consequence of agreeing a legal contract, but was already present because our ancestors lived together in small communities.

Humans can be egotistical and selfish, but that should not blind us to the fact that social behaviour is also programmed by nature. Characteristics such as care and cooperation are dominant in our evolutionary processes.[2] We share these traits with our nearest family members, the great apes, and they go back to our common ancestor, which must have lived around five to eight million years ago. As proof of this, De Waal uses his observations to show that primates have many characteristics closely linked with human morality: sympathy, empathy, altruism, friendship and the capacity to set arguments aside. According to De Waal, animals help each other in ways that may even run counter to their self-interest, which means that something abstract like moral awareness is not the preserve of humans. Contrary to proponents of the social contract, such as Hobbes, who start with a conception of humans as fundamentally asocial or even antisocial creatures, De Waal claims that we are naturally social and empathetic. Or to put it simply, the human species is an empathic herd animal with a strong sense of community spirit.

Infectious yawning

The question is how big or small the gap between humans and animals is. How human are animals, and how bestial are humans? In other words, is it possible to draw a sharp line between us and other animals? No, says De Waal. He speaks of an emotional continuum with other animals, particularly the primates that are our nearest relatives, consisting of three different levels of morality. The first and second levels of this continuum reveal a great deal of overlap with primates. Only the third layer of morality is exclusive to humans. He uses the image of traditional Russian matryoshka dolls, each containing a smaller doll, which in turn contains a smaller one. De Waal takes a broad definition of morality, which he sees as a system of rules and incentives for solving rivalry and conflicts within the group. By this definition, morality is closely related to social behaviour and comprises positive traits such as altruism, helpfulness and care, which constrain our behaviour, especially when conflict arises between members of a group due to misaligned interests. In *The Age of Empathy*, published in 2009, he uses the term empathy to cover concern for the other and the desire to help.

The first level of morality is comprised of moral feelings. Empathy belongs here, as does reciprocity, retribution, conflict resolution and a sense of fairness. Empathy is an exceptionally difficult concept to pin down, but I will follow De Waal in saying that it is about understanding and sharing one another's feelings. In order to do this, it is necessary to be able to imagine yourself in another person's position. It is a form of bond between individuals that precedes language and is beautifully expressed in German as *Einfühlung*. Imitation and infection are important related processes. For instance, we tend to imitate other people's movements: when you see someone yawn, you do it too. Empathy plays an important role in this process. Scientists believe that yawning along with someone is a way of maintaining a social relationship with them. Yawning at the sight of another person's yawn begins around the age of five, when children grow better at observing the emotions of others and understanding the feelings behind certain behaviour. Children already yawn in the womb, as do other animals, from chimpanzees to dogs.

According to De Waal, emotional infectiousness – taking on the emotional state of another – is an automatic reflex exhibited by both humans and animals. Taking care of another person is the next step, including behaviours such as comforting among primates. Elephants, wolves and some corvids, specifically ravens and rooks, exhibit comforting behaviour. For instance, Indian elephants comfort one another when they're upset by moving their trunks towards one another's faces and making sounds. In doing so, they take on the posture and mood of the affected elephant. De Waal refers to the highest level of empathy as perspective-taking, which makes it possible to give targeted help to another. Offering help requires emotional involvement, understanding of the situation and the ability to come up with a solution. Other animal species are also capable of this, including the great apes, elephants and cetaceans.

Researchers have identified a fitting illustration of the first level of morality in bonobos, who shared the kill from their hunt with 'strangers'. The primatologists saw a male bonobo in the forests of Congo capture a type of antelope and take it high up a tree to eat it. In response, nine bonobo females also climbed the tree, five from his own group and four from another. The females from his own group used arm gestures and sounds to indicate that he should share the meat – among bonobos females are dominant and occupy the top of the group social structure. Conflicts in the group are solved by sharing food and by lots of sex. In reaction to the loud exhortations of the nine females, the five females from his own group and one from the other group were granted a piece of meat by the male bonobo. The male then allowed the female from the other group to take the antelope's head and share it with the females from both groups.[3]

The second level of morality relates to the social pressure exerted on every member of a community 'to contribute to common goals and uphold agreed-upon social rules', De Waal writes.[4] At this level, we find the first differences from our closest relatives. Chimpanzees may also distinguish between acceptable and unacceptable behaviour, but they mainly make this distinction with respect to themselves and focus on the direct consequences of the behaviour exhibited. Among animals, communal interests are rather less of a priority than among humans. The situations where this does become an issue usually involve high-ranking chimpanzees putting an end to fights. This behaviour is seen among chimpanzees both in the wild and in captivity. De Waal writes that in this case, the group as a whole benefits from the peace-making of the high-ranking chimpanzees, because it 'enhances social cohesion and cooperation'.[5]

At the third level of morality, comparisons with other animals are scarce. This level is about moral judgement and reasoning. Only humans, De Waal notes, follow an inner compass, a consistent internal moral framework, and judge themselves and others, taking into account the intentions and convictions behind their behaviour. While animals in their moral behaviour are primarily motivated by their emotions, humans elevate their behaviour and that of others to a level of abstraction where we attempt to apply a certain logic. This means that humans can rationalise the way they should behave in particular circumstances based on templates such as good and evil, reaching beyond the empathy mentioned above. Humans express their moral approval or disapproval of situations, even when they themselves are not participants. This is the major difference between morality among humans and animals.

The banality of good

De Waal is not alone in his criticism of Hobbes. Other authors are critical of the Hobbesian view of humans as bestial animals and point out that every day we commit countless acts of solidarity and helpfulness, which have a major influence on the quality of our contact with others. Humans can do terrible things to one another, but if you take a level-headed look at our lives, we naturally do a great deal of good every day; it is just so normal that it is quickly forgotten. The banality of good, you might call it, with a nod to Hannah Arendt. In his 2015 work *Altruism*, for instance, Buddhist philosopher Matthieu Ricard, son of the famous French philosopher Jean-François Revel, rejects the assumption that humans are egotistical monsters through and through, naturally inclined towards violence and rivalry, and exclusively focused on pursuing their personal interests.[6] Based on countless studies, Ricard claims that there is little or no scientific evidence for the violent nature of humans. Of course humans commit violent acts – they murder and rob their way through history – but according to Ricard, it is a historical fallacy to categorise all such behaviour, which generally remains restricted to personal conflicts, in terms of ubiquitous war. With Hobbes's assumptions in mind, Ricard notes that we should abandon our belief in humans being brutal, bloodthirsty and instinctively violent. Nature does not revolve around conflict and aggression, but rather, as Ricard concurs with De Waal, around cooperation and peaceful co-existence.

As an extension of this, other critical minds express a desire to appeal more to our empathic feelings and point out that individual and collective violence has continuously decreased over the last thousand years, and quite particularly remarkably in the past sixty years. Despite countless brutal conflicts, on a worldwide basis there has been a spectacular drop in institutionalised forms of violence (such as cruel punishments, slavery and executions), everyday violence against vulnerable groups such as women, children, animals and homosexual people, and violence in the form of wars and ethnic cleansing. In his famous book *The Better Angels of Our Nature*, published in 2011, evolutionary psychologist Steven Pinker attributes this reduction in violence to various causes, including a growing emphasis on human rationality, increased moral sensibility, feminisation of society and a stronger emphasis on empathy. While De Waal emphasises that empathy is a neurologically and evolutionarily rooted effect, Pinker claims that it springs from identification with the other – and so is a 'reflective affect'.[7]

In *Together*, Richard Sennett makes an instructive distinction between sympathy (a 'hot' response) and empathy (a 'cold' response).[8] While sympathy takes sides and identifies with someone, empathy gives free rein to curiosity about the other, to dialogue, openness and the possibility of other (non-violent) directions for a resolution. Australian cultural philosopher Roman Krznaric works this idea out further in his 2014 book *Empathy*, when he argues that empathy creates human bonds that make life worth living. He makes an impassioned plea for a true revolution in human relations, with the aim of acquiring new habits such as 'outrospection', so that we look inwards less and outwards more, towards the other. Krznaric even goes so far as to argue for an empathy museum, envisaged as a playground where people can enter into spiritual fusion.

The plea for more empathy sounds nice, so much is irrefutable, yet there has also been a sharp backlash. When empathising you also need to watch out, as Johnny Rotten makes clear in the song by his group Public Image Ltd.: 'This is not a love song / No, no, no, no.' You need to pay attention to avoid allowing empathy to deteriorate into revelling under the pretext of 'make love, not war'. Many positive philosophical mantras forget that aggressive expressions are also part of life and have their uses. Moreover, how does the empathetic revolution relate to real action? Is empathy actually a useful tool for policy makers and politicians? When charity becomes the guiding principle, as American psychologist Paul Bloom and Belgian philosopher Ignaas Devisch see it, chances are we will not get very far.[9] Empathy alone is insufficient to solve major social problems. Worse still, Krznaric's empathy revolution can stand in the way of structural change. If we really want to go a different way, then we need more than personal involvement and our own fuzzy feelings. The problem is that with empathy we focus our attention specifically on the situation of a particular person or that of a group from our own biotope. In reality we largely grant empathy to people with whom we identify and in whom we recognise ourselves. The further someone is from us, the less empathy we feel for them. For that reason, Bloom argues for taking care of other people and trying to improve their situation without feeling their emotions oneself. Rational compassion, as he puts it.

Take care of each other

According to De Waal, security is the main reason for every form of social life, and it arises through cooperation and having a sharp eye for others' physical and psychological needs. That is not how we normally view security. In Western history, the concept 'security' is grafted onto the meaning of the Latin word *securitas*, which consists of the three elements *se* ('without'), *cura* ('care') and *tas* (a state of 'being'). The political and theoretical meaning of the word refers to the Pax Romana, the Roman peace, which lasted more than two hundred years and was personified as a female figure. In medieval times, the term *securitas* was used to express the protection of life and property within the national state. That resulted in a dual image. On the one hand it was about protection of streets, squares and markets. In these places you needed government protection against citizens with malicious intentions. On the other hand, *securitas* stood for something we would now call defence: the protection of a state or country against external powers.

From the moment in the second half of the 20th century when crime and disorder substantially increased in the Western world, the citizen began to feel more readily insecure. We have become so socialised to talk in negative terms about security, that talking about security really boils down to talking about insecurity. You might also say that insecurity and security are synonyms, more or less interchangeable concepts. In an experiment you can try out yourself, ask someone what 'security' means, and they will talk about how insecure we are and why crime should be more robustly dealt with. Only those who have never been attacked or suffered a break-in are deemed secure. In his 2013 philological study *Security*, John Hamilton shows that this is a tenuous definition of security. In his view, security is much more than the absence of crime and disorder, which is indicated by the etymology of the word *cura*. *Cura* in the Latin word *securitas* has dual meanings. Being 'free of care' can mean living without turmoil or fear, a definition that takes us back to Hobbes's negative image of humanity, described above, whereby security is understood as the elimination of 'pain' or 'danger' (*se-cura*). In this view, *cura* refers to anything that can cause turmoil, and humans are only secure when their lives are devoid of 'pain' or 'danger'. But, Hamilton continues, *cura* can also be positively explained, in terms of 'attentiveness' and 'diligence'. In this sense, it is a form of care that you bestow upon something or someone; *cura* is 'care for an object' as well as being 'an object of care' in itself. This meaning of *securitas* is relevant to this chapter. From this we can derive the idea that 'care' must be offered in order to live 'free of care'. The positive meaning of security shines through.

The insight that security encompasses more than the negative criterion of being 'free of care' chimes with a deeper intuition, which can also be read in the etymology of the Dutch word *veiligheid* (security). *Veiligheid* is originally derived from the Middle Dutch *velich* and Old Frisian *felig*. The meanings of the two words involve being 'without danger', but also point to 'loyalty', 'trustworthiness' and 'friendliness'. The same aspects of meaning are also central to the German word *Geborgenheit* and the Swedish *trygghet*, words which are generally translated into English as 'security'. Swedish *trygghet*, however, has more positive connotations than security, because it points to meanings such as 'trust' and 'attachment to society'. German *Geborgenheit* is also primarily about the feeling that you're in a place which offers shelter and protection. Feeling at home, for instance, a 'sense of belonging', as we put it in English, invokes a feeling of security, as does the extent of your connection with the neighbourhood where you live and your relationships with other residents. Giving and receiving trust within a communal space where people feel comfortable and as if they belong, are important aspects of these European words for security.

It will be clear that Hobbes's selfish human image and De Waal's social human vision set out above are at odds. It is in this very tension between them that security gains a negative and a positive meaning, without the two meanings becoming diametrically opposed. Nevertheless, some correction is required to the prevailing idea that an exclusively negative human image lies at the foundation of security. If this misconception persists, then thinking around security will be dogged by the assumption of an original civil war. To put it another way: although the use of the term 'security' in the sense of crime and disorder is not incorrect, this perspective requires supplementation. Security has two aspects: one negative and one positive. The negative aspect is characterised by surveillance, control and zero tolerance to combat insecurity. The positive aspect of security is much more about matters such as offering care and trust. That means that combating insecurity ('negative security') is fundamentally different from creating security ('positive security'). Positive security requires different language, and different tools than repressive instruments and the business-like social contract. In other words, how can you think about security without resorting to police?

Peace, security and health

Attention for positive security has not simply been plucked out of thin air. In international politics since the end of the 1960s, there has been a prominent change of course towards more positive ways of improving security. This change began when the Norwegian sociologist Johan Galtung developed a positive and a negative concept of peace, and researched the relationship between the two.[10] In Galtung's view, negative peace means an end to war, so that there is no further armed conflict between or within states. Positive peace, by contrast, refers to a condition free of violence, one of sustainability and justice. In this distinction, Galtung expresses criticism of the assumption that peace is nothing more than the absence of war and armed conflict, as it was during the Pax Romana. Positive peace is about much more: it demands attention for a stable economy, sufficient food and clean drinking water, a sound education system, properly functioning democratic institutions and so on. Galtung drew his inspiration for this distinction between positive and negative peace from medical science, where 'health' refers both to the absence of disease and to the ways in which the body can withstand illness.

Internationally, there has also been a growing realisation that something precedes security, namely conditions that make people feel safe. With the end of the Cold War, the world entered a new era. Breaking the ice between Reagan and Gorbachev and the thawing of relations between the two countries in the 1980s meant that international military conflicts no longer represented the greatest threat to the security of the individual. After the 'phase of political hysteria', as Saul

Bellow termed the Cold War in a letter to President Dwight D. Eisenhower as recorded in his famous 1964 novel *Herzog*, other problems make it onto the agenda, demanding concrete solutions: climate change, environmental issues, social inequality, health risks, hunger and poverty. The United Nations refers to all of this as 'human security', a term that springs from the UN's ambition to do more about basic human living conditions. That demonstrates political courage, but also good sense. Instead of opting for reactive military policy to attain freedom by ending conflicts, security should be much more about peacebuilding and working on factors with a positive effect on security. That is not to say that military intervention is not sometimes needed to protect citizens in life-threatening situations, but according to the UN, investing in peace works better. In doing this, people can develop optimally and enjoy their freedom.

It is not just the words that change; actions shift with them. Though it is difficult to provide an exhaustive list of all positive factors of human security, in a nutshell, the UN needs to tackle issues such as unclean drinking water, unstable economies, homelessness, violation of human rights, pollution, ethnic tensions and domestic violence. In the 2003 report *Human Security – Now,* two strategies are mentioned for tackling these: protection and empowerment. Protection involves the nation states taking the lead in protecting citizens against threats over which they have no control, such as unclean drinking water, while empowerment appeals to people's own potential and asks them to dedicate their efforts to the improvement of their lives and environment. What is striking is that the focus shifts from thinking in terms of shortcomings to people's own capacity and that of their broader environment to change things for the better. The self-organising side of society plays a major role in this new perspective. In other words, the power of the community becomes central, instead of the might of the state.

One problem with this is that in essence, the concept 'human security' is still about eliminating threats in order to live a happy and healthy life. The term remains fixed in a negative definition. In his study *Security, Identity, Interests*, sociologist Bill McSweeney therefore links the relational aspects of security with the new focus in international politics.[11] International security, after all, is not primarily about danger or threats, nor is it about the means of preventing or tackling them, but about the question of how we can create the right conditions for society to flourish. Nevertheless, this last question is often ignored, because we tend to pay attention mainly to what endangers societies instead of what makes people happy and connects them. In order to think more positively about security, McSweeney, like Galtung, points to the analogy with what we understand under 'health'. Our tendency to talk of health in terms of 'not being ill' means we are mainly focused on eliminating causes of diseases instead of paying attention to what makes us healthy. Healing is not the key aspect of health; at its heart are issues such as healthy eating and fitness, and basic conditions such as hygiene and education.[12] Strangely enough, healthcare is much less focused on the sustainability of our health, although all policy documents are currently teeming with the word 'sustainable'.

Positive places

Security is a dual concept. You can interpret it negatively, as combating crime and disorder, but you can also interpret it positively, as offering care and trust. In policy terms, this means that alongside the negative definition – trying to protect citizens from something – security can also be understood in a more inclusive, affirmative manner. In the latter case, it is a matter of protection by each other instead of focusing on how people can best be protected against each other. In concrete terms, this can involve positive role models, from sports, music, dance, fashion or religion, which can serve as mentors to young people at risk in vulnerable neighbourhoods. Or it could mean initiatives such as the 'Positive Tickets' project in Vancouver, where, besides fines, police officers hand out vouchers to reward good behaviour by young people. The vouchers can be exchanged for an ice-cream or a swim. The Miami police are doing something similar under the slogan 'Do the Right Thing'. Young people who wear a helmet when cycling or help elderly people cross a busy road are rewarded with a free slice of pizza. Closer to home, informal meeting places on a district level in the Netherlands offer care and safety to residents, as in the case of the Leeszaal (The Reading Room) and De Woonkamer van Meneer de Burgemeester (The Mayor's Living Room) in Rotterdam.

De Leeszaal Rotterdam West was founded in 2013 on Rijnhoutplein behind Nieuwe Binnenweg, the longest shopping street in the Netherlands. A favourite meeting place for neighbourhood residents, the place is run by more than eighty volunteers, who organise language classes, children's programmes, poetry evenings, debates and book launches there. The initiative was launched by two residents, out of frustration that communal spaces such as the library, local community centres and an education centre had been closed by the local authority. Not far from the Leeszaal we find another initiative, De Woonkamer. De Woonkamer is on Burgemeester Meineszlaan, in the Nieuwe Westen district, an area with more than 19,000 residents from many different cultures. Residents here organise easily accessible activities, from film mornings to discussion evenings. One day you could attend a French lesson, another a clothing swap. You also encounter local officials here: employees of the security department of the municipal authority have their offices here, so that local residents can more easily contact the municipality with questions or problems.

De Leeszaal and De Woonkamer are the ideal image of positive security. They are examples of social infrastructure in action, shared spaces where people can assemble and can get to know one another. As such, they are local spots bringing positive change to the security in the neighbourhood. By joining forces and collaborating, the residents easily come into contact with one another, leading to reduced prejudice and increased tolerance. Trust and care begin very locally, with your neighbour, your street, your district. Residents receive a lesson in diversity by meeting people from different backgrounds as well as coming to identify more with the neighbourhood, increasing social control. Local places reinforce public familiarity in a neighbourhood, which in turn influences residents' sense of security and their faith in government. On a deeper level, these bubble breakers respond to a primal sense of safety, which has come under considerable pressure in the neoliberal context of loss of solidarity and over-individualisation. Neoliberalism has blind faith in the Sacred Market. It preaches freedom and open borders and has led to up-scaling beyond recognition, a situation no one asked for. Neoliberalism has blurred the picture of who we are and where we belong, damaging the remaining sense of community citizens still feel or want to restore. There is ever less space in our society for community or communal identity. Many citizens feel uprooted and uncomfortable as a result, something I address in more detail in Chapter 7. This is referred to as the opposition between *sense of space* and *sense of place*. Sense of space indicates the measurable space, sense of place the perceived space, feeling at home in a particular place and the sense of belonging somewhere.

Particularly in super-diverse districts, where the original population has become one of the minority groups, the challenge is to get citizens to the point where they pay more attention to one another and engage in socially relevant activities together. For not only do the residents of these districts feel less secure, crime also increases because the social connections in the neighbourhood break down – and with them social control. It is easy to talk about 'social cohesion', but actually increasing that cohesion in a given district is extremely difficult. Social cohesion is based on trust between people, which is necessarily a voluntary process. As a government you cannot just say, 'Go forth and trust one another.' Moreover, in these districts citizens' faith in government is at a historical low. In various districts in South Rotterdam, for instance, figures for trust in government have dropped below 50%. We see the same trend in comparable districts in other Western cities, where the stubborn problems of our society continue to accumulate, including unemployment, medical problems and illiteracy. Here, too, trust and satisfaction towards the government is at a very low ebb.

At first glance, trust correlates with rational, evidence-based indicators such as the number of reports the police write each week. But ask residents what trust means to them and you receive a completely different answer. Trust is not so much to do with the objective performance of the police, but with the human sides of police behaviour, with the perception of the processes that culminate in their performance. Confidence in the police is most often dented when police action is perceived as unfair. Discrimination, intimidation and excessive use of violence all impair trust in the police. Recent examples of this are ethnic profiling and a policy of targeting youths with conspicuously expensive possessions such as coats or fast cars. For instance, in the Netherlands there was a great deal of commotion about the interrogation of rapper Typhoon, because his profile (i.e. skin colour) did not fit with the expensive car he was driving. Police violence against minorities also sharpens the debate on the street, rather than contributing to greater trust among citizens in police action.

I will not claim that more attention for positive security will automatically increase social cohesion and cause crime to melt away, but it makes sense to me for security professionals to take a closer look at new ways of putting non-punitive government resources to work. In recent years, security policy seems to have headed down a dead-end street of more repression in a way that defies common sense. There are more positive ways of creating security, though these would require the government to take on a different role. The transformation towards positive change in security on a district level is not just about citizens taking the initiative, but also about the government aligning itself with such initiatives. When given access to real resources, communities often have good ideas about how to reduce crime through nonpunitive mechanisms, as sociologist Alex Vitale shows in his 2017 book *The End of Policing*. Local spots which make the city into a village often only arise when the municipal authorities lend those taking the initiative a helping hand, for instance by removing red tape such as complex procedures that take many years to complete. Reducing bureaucracy is sadly more often the exception than the rule. Many municipalities still think that detailed regulations and painstaking checks result in greater security. But however unlikely it might sound, security can also benefit from fewer rules.

Phantom security

It is hard to fight hysteria. As long as politicians believe that threatening war and destruction works, even in the face of consistent evidence to the contrary, they will continue to serve up hysterical, warlike language. Politicians understand better than anyone that such exaggerated language is an effective political tool for speaking about security. Hysteria leads to popular attention; everyone is swept along, while the soft language of connection and trust is boring by contrast. Furthermore, it is seen in a bad light due to associations with subsidies and benefits, and a culture of pampering. In practice, 'connection' and 'trust' are also concepts without a clearly delineated meaning, which makes them difficult to measure and to capture in bureaucratic procedures.

The enormous overproduction of rules and regulations therefore continues to exist, as does the exaggerated effort of combating evil. I have termed this 'security hysteria'. American trainee police officers, for instance, are taught to fire weapons and apprehend suspects, not to seek contact with people they encounter in the street. A study by the Police Executive Research Forum revealed that trainees as a rule received 58 hours of instruction on firearms, 49 hours on self-defence, 10 hours on communication skills and 8 hours on de-escalation tactics. Compare this with conflict resolution among primates: after a conflict the warring factions come together for reconciliation, by embracing, kissing, grooming or having sex. The Dutch word for reconciliation, *verzoenen* comes from Middle High German *süene*, which means 'mediation', 'peace' or 'kiss'. The Dutch word *zoen* came to mean 'kiss' because reconciliation was often sealed with a kiss.

You do not win any wars with hysteria. In other words, you cannot enforce understanding of public affairs through rules, punishments and bludgeoning alone. Too much emphasis on combating crime leads to increased feelings of insecurity and reduced trust in government – all that while in many Western countries, things have never been so secure as they are now. While Hobbes's point of departure was to establish a state that would eliminate fear of crime, disorder and victimhood, that very same fear is now encouraged by a state which implements all kinds of control and surveillance measures without restraint. To me it seems that we are dealing with 'phantom security', by which I mean the phenomenon of improvements in security leading to more insecurity. Or, to put it simply, hysterically trying to tackle any form of insecurity leads to precisely the opposite outcome. You continue to see insecurity everywhere, even when it is safer than ever. A good example of this is the rise of vigilantes and neighbourhood watch groups in European countries such as Belgium and Germany. Anyone who deviates from the norm, from loitering groups of youths to dark-skinned young men with beards, runs a high risk of being accosted by these teams, who dress in bullet-proof, stab-proof vests and use drones, professional flashlights and infrared cameras – and in a few cases even a fully equipped command vehicle. The surprising thing is, you generally see them in relatively safe districts, and not in deprived areas, where you would really expect them.

The government promises security, but makes things surprisingly insecure. This paradox also becomes apparent when we look at trust in government intervention, an important condition for a secure society. German sociologist Niklas Luhmann speaks of trust in terms of a strategy for reducing social complexity, a way of simplifying life and dealing with risks and uncertainty, while simultaneously assuming that a positive future will become reality.[13] In *The Burnout Society*, published in 2015, Korean-German philosopher Byung-Chul Han emphasises that this is about building up a positive relationship with the other, even when we do not know that other person personally. Thus trust in the government leads to a greater willingness among residents to comply with rules and to collaborate with the government, for instance tipping off the police about people trying to radicalise others in the area. Moreover, trust reinforces the legitimacy of police action in the district and increases the sense of security. A precondition for this is that citizens are treated with respect. People's feeling of safety is strongly associated with a sense of being fairly treated and the government making it clear that they belong.

You only get trust when you can give it, and building trust is particularly important in super-diverse districts. The more diverse the neighbourhood, the more complicated it is to live together. Social tensions can run high, and security problems are often serious. A complicating factor here is that many residents of these neighbourhoods have serious doubts about the fairness of police action, even when their own experiences with neighbourhood officers are good. For instance, ethnic minorities have less confidence in the police than the majority. They're also more sensitive to issues such as unequal treatment and intimidation by the police than the indigenous population, for whom 'belonging' is much less of an issue. It also transpires that trust is dented when discrimination and excessive use of force become the topic of the day in the media. Repressive tools such as ethnic profiling and targeting conspicuous wealth can therefore be counterproductive. They add tension to the relationship between police and the people in the street, leading to greater feelings of insecurity and reduced confidence in the police. These issues, which follow from breaking off the social relationship between government and citizen, can form fertile ground for hysteria, as I show in Chapter 6.

Moreover, and that is the second remarkable point, security measures often have a completely different effect than is originally intended, even in completely different areas. The original aim of such a measure shifts insidiously, as it is applied to purposes it was never meant for. A particular measure may be proportionate in particular circumstances, but that does not exclude the possibility of the same measure becoming disproportionate when applied simultaneously or sequentially in completely different circumstances, whether the difference is the person to whom it is applied or in the effectiveness of the approach. A distressing illustration of this is the abuse of anti-terrorism legislation, which allows investigative authorities to monitor phone and internet traffic without democratic control. For instance, in the UK the Regulation of Investigatory Powers Act came into force in 2000, making it easier for the intelligence services and the police to place citizens under surveillance if they were suspected of terrorist activities. Internet traffic can be intercepted without permission from a judge. But the law is also used by small local authorities for completely difference activities. The English town of Workington struggles with a plague of pigeons, and under this law the local authority monitors citizens they suspect of feeding the birds. The town of Bromley uses the law to keep an eye on 'antisocial' citizens, and Lincoln to prevent sale of cigarettes and alcohol to minors. In Caerphilly, a town in south Wales, they track illegal tattoo artists on the same grounds. In the Scottish county of Midlothian, the national antiterrorist law is used to combat barking dogs, and in Wolverhampton they use it to keep tabs on the sale of dangerous toys.

This kind of abuse of powers visibly undermines support from society for new security measures. The approach to serious problems such as terrorism also leads to a culture of control that has got completely out of hand, with security measures being drawn up against an endless variety of effectively trivial risks, such as dangerous toys and barking dogs. The security approach thus has precisely the opposite of the intended effect: it increases insecurity. That is how phantom security works, like a pyromaniac firefighter.

Conclusion

Security is never found in isolation. On the one hand there are the ideas of philosophers such as Hobbes, who start out from a negative interpretation of security coupled with a chaotic state of nature. Under this view, the police force and criminal law are the main tools for preventing a fierce 'war of all against all'. This means that combating crime takes the form of a government threatening potential culprits with punishment if they break the law. Violence or the threat of violence by the government is needed to avoid falling back into an original human state of violence. The view of humanity behind this reduces humans to dangerous creatures, malicious by nature, motivated by negative emotions such as fear and hate. All sorts of projected fears have made security a national obsession, and the language of security has gained a strong resemblance to a hysterical hyperbole machine, bringing the feared reality closer. It is like fighting fire with fire.

On the other hand, the insights of De Waal and Ricard present a more positive view of humanity, within which there is space for empathy, compassion and altruism. In his scientific publications and popular books, De Waal makes it clear that automatic empathy is activated in both humans and animals when they see one of their species in pain. This capacity probably arose early in evolution and leads to the protection of people from one's own group in cases of need. This means that humans are primarily social creatures and only operate as individuals as a secondary function. They live at least as much alongside others and thanks to others as they do for themselves. This notion that humans need others and community for their existence and fulfilment allows more space for the importance of mutual protection; this contrasts with perspectives focused primarily on how humans can best protect themselves against one another's egocentric and violent impulses.

According to Hobbes, fear brings people together, but of course the opposite is also true: trust brings people together just as well. Shared urban spaces as the Leeszaal and De Woonkamer van Meneer de Burgemeester – 'palaces for the people', as sociologist Eric Klinenberg would call them – allow people to make connections, help one another, and offer refuge to those who feel excluded or diminished elsewhere. It seems to me that both the positive and the negative sides of security create a reality, and that the two realities co-exist. Or to put it differently, not everything revolves around combating insecurity, pulling up weeds; it is also a matter of planting and promoting the positive factors of community, such as care, trust and cooperation. There is every reason to reinforce positive security, because the negative approach in practice contributes to a strange and unproductive paradox. Security policy and the hysterical rhetoric used for it represent an ever greater obstacle to increased security – phantom security, as I have termed it. That does not change the fact that serious crime must be dealt with, but it means that security and insecurity are subject to completely different laws. The concept 'security' is fundamentally split. For that reason, in this chapter I have presented an understanding of security and insecurity as two separate realities. When the emphasis shifts from a negative to a positive view of security, the starting point changes, and with it the methods applied. The use of different terms for security is much more than a matter of switching name tags. Positive security requires a different vocabulary and a new toolkit.

Notes

1 De Waal (2006, p. 5).
2 Biologists point out that nature relies on various forms of collaboration. For instance, there are all kinds of tiny creatures in the intestines of cockroaches and in the rumens of goats and cattle. According to researchers, ocean life also revolves around other forms of relationship between species than merely competition. The driving force here is not survival of the fittest, but collaboration. Coral, for example, needs algae to convert sunlight into energy, and those algae in turn live in the coral. Some biologists therefore go a step further and argue that nature is not about the strongest individuals surviving but the strongest system, which depends on collaboration and support rather than competition.
3 'Bonobos Also Share their Kill with "Strangers"', *NRC Handelsblad*, 7 April 2018.
4 De Waal (2006, p. 169).
5 De Waal (2006, p. 171).
6 Thinking on altruism has a long sociological history that can be traced through the work of Auguste Comte, Peter Kropotkin, Émile Durkheim, Marcel Mauss and Pierre Bourdieu among others. In his work *The Divison of Labor in Society*, Durkheim links altruism with solidarity: 'Wherever there are societies, there is altruism, because there is solidarity' (Durkheim 1960, p. 215). Kropotkin described the propensity of both animals and man to help one another and called this reciprocal altruism 'mutual aid'.
7 Oosterling (2013, p. 378).
8 Sennett (2012).
9 Bloom (2016); Devisch (2017).
10 Galtung (1969).
11 McSweeney (1999).
12 Similarly, positive psychology considers how people can thrive. According to the leading exponents of this movement, Martin Seligman and Mihaly Csikszentmihalyi, traditional clinical psychology focuses too much on weak points ('What's wrong with you?') and too little on strengths ('What's right with you?'). In other words, it is not primarily about what is wrong in our heads, but about what makes our lives worth living. For that reason this movement focuses not only on repairing what has gone wrong – phobias, trauma, depression – but is particularly occupied with reinforcing positive experiences and qualities in people, such as happiness, pleasure, wellbeing, friendship, empathy and love (Seligman & Csikszentmihalyi, 2000). Focusing exclusively on negative emotions does not do justice to the fullness of life.
13 Luhmann (2000).

Chapter 5

From *Minority Report* to reporting minorities

Introduction

In the key scene of the episode 'Nosedive' from the British science fiction series *Black Mirror*, the mildly hysterical main character, a young woman named Lacie Pound, discovers that she needs a social rating above 4.5 to move to the attractive Pelican Cove Lifestyle Community. According to her estate agent, a score like that would get her a 20% discount on her dream apartment. The personal score is calculated from judgements on a scale of 1 to 5 by other characters, including passers-by, friends and colleagues. Socially desirable behaviour, such as showing appreciation for others, gets you a higher rating. Interaction with people with a higher rating also raises Lacie's score. Using special contact lenses which project that contextual information onto her retina, Lacie immediately sees the ratings of people around her and can also give them points for their behaviour.

Black Mirror is a series about the excesses of technology and modern communications media. Shane Allen, head of comedy at the BBC, describes the series as 'satirical drama for the social media generation'. The title *Black Mirror* refers to the screen of the television or mobile when switched off. The compelling thing about the episode 'Nosedive' is the way Lacie, an ambitious woman in her thirties, is so obsessed with her rating that she will do anything to get as high a score as possible. A high score offers a great many privileges. If you want luxury accommodation in a gated community or to dine in the better restaurants, you have to attain at least a 4.5, but if you come in under 2.5, you're part of the social underclass. Failing to achieve 4.5, Lacie misses out on her dream apartment, and due to all kinds of unfortunate events, her score continues to drop. She gradually descends to the grey and grimy dregs of society and eventually ends up in prison, broken and tired, but relieved that she is finally somewhere where she can say what she thinks and how she feels, far away from a hysterical society in which everyone is constantly preoccupied judging the behaviour of others on Facebook, Twitter and Instagram.

The makers of *Black Mirror* cannot predict the exact future, but *Black Mirror* is certainly a series that in outlining an image of the future provides commentary on the things we currently take for granted. The dark side of the scoring of people based on their behaviour is in fact never far away when it comes to Facebook, Twitter and Instagram. Originally, social media functioned as a sort of public space, a place for connection and informal meeting between people from different social backgrounds and positions. This point of departure has changed slowly but surely in recent years. The nature of social media is anything but social these days, as everyone now competes and compares themselves with others. Rather than open fora where arguments and information are freely exchanged, Facebook, Twitter and Instagram are platforms for competition and longing for status; digital reward systems where everything revolves around acquiring as many followers, likes and retweets as possible.

Our behaviour on social media is a typical hysterical phenomenon. Lots of people have completely lost control over the amount of time they spend on social media. We spend more time each day on Facebook than eating. We're constantly tagging, posting, following, spamming, liking and scoring people on the basis of their behaviour. There are plenty of positive aspects to this; for instance, a reputation score on the internet, an online evaluation of a person or company, is a quick way of gaining insight into someone far away whom you do not know. Take eBay, for example, which works by an ingenious valuation system to keep purchase and sale of articles on the right tracks. But while it offers a better service to customers, more efficient and lower costs, it is easy to forget that the technology that makes this possible also enables mass surveillance and can lead to thought police who come to arrest you even before you have done anything.

'This is what you'll get when you mess with us'

When you start to pay attention, you soon see that predicting behaviour through scoring people is gaining ever broader application. The Chinese government is working on a national social credit system that allocates every Chinese citizen – all 1.4 billion – a score based on his or her behavioural traits, varying from financial credit-worthiness to driving offences and from behaviour on social media to dog walking. Details of the precise functioning of the credit scores remain vague, but it is clear that by collecting large quantities of data, the trustworthiness of citizens will be mapped. The data come from the police, financial institutions, the government and internet companies such as the e-commerce site Alibaba, the search engine Baidu and the social media branch of Tencent. Citizens also have an active role in this new scoring system, in evaluating their teachers or doctors. Points are deducted for activities such as gambling and for having a criminal record. By contrast, paying off a bank loan or buying nappies is rewarded with bonus points, because it points to responsible behaviour.

As in *Black Mirror*, a low credit score in China has far-reaching consequences. Citizens can be excluded from certain jobs, accommodation or loans and have only restricted access to the internet. On the other hand, people with a high citizen score enjoy a number of advantages, including easier access to travel visas, hospitals and subsidies. The introduction of the refined scoring system is the result of the blurring of moral standards in Chinese society. The institute responsible for its development states that China has changed in recent years from a society of acquaintances into a society of strangers. In order to expand social control according to the institute, an evaluation system is needed to control and guide the behaviour of Chinese residents, more extensively and more precisely than was the case under Mao.

The Chinese system, which objectifies and ranks its residents into A-, B-, C- or D-citizens, sounds Orwellian, or at least like a bizarre description of life in a completely over-controlled society. But predicting behaviour and attributing points to it is also at work in our neoliberal society; it is simply differently packaged. Companies such as Facebook and Google collect as much data as possible about people in order to influence them through targeted advertisements. Based on your profile, the algorithms of Amazon and Netflix ensure that you no longer have to think about what book to buy or film to watch. They save you the stress of choosing from the enormous range of books and films, because they make the best choice there is based on your online behaviour. Do you watch *Black Mirror?* Then you might also like the movie *The Circle.* Harvard professor Shoshana Zuboff speaks of the surveillance capitalist nightmare, in which everything revolves around consumer scores and access to digital platforms.[1] According to the World Privacy Forum, there are now thousands of different consumer scores. You already have one if you have a bank account. The same goes for buying a plane ticket. On the website Rate My Professor you can score lecturers. A certain Robert Campbell scores 3.5 – he's a 'terrifying, strange, psychotic man', according to an accompanying comment.

Using new technologies to monitor and analyse people's behaviour also changes many aspects of combating crime. Investigative agencies are attempting to use large-scale smart data-analyses to gain an idea of whether our behaviour indicates criminal activity. The aim is to predict where and when a crime might be committed, as well as by whom. The British intelligence service GCHQ, one of the best and most aggressive intelligence services in the world, does some of the better oracle work by collecting data from internet users from more than 185 countries, including the United States, England, Ireland, Canada, Mexico, Spain, France, Germany and the Netherlands. The system GCHQ uses is called Karma Police, after the Radiohead song of the same name, in which Thom Yorke sings, 'This is what you'll get / When you mess with us.' Documents and files leaked by the whistleblower Edward Snowden have revealed that GCHQ uses cookies from Google, Yahoo, Facebook, Reddit, WordPress, Hotmail and CNN, among others. Visits to the porn site YouPorn are also recorded. Not only is the browser history of internet users analysed, but e-mail, chat and search engine data are also collected and stored under separate user profiles. In 2012, around fifty billion units of metadata were collected a day, and GCHQ wants to increase this to one hundred billion. All this is justified under the organisation's legal task of protecting the wellbeing of the United Kingdom.

In the Netherlands too, predictive policing, predicting crime based on large quantities of data, is no longer a matter for the distant future. In fact, the Netherlands is at the forefront internationally, as the first country in the world to predict on a national level where and when crime will be committed. In other countries, including the United States and Britain, this currently only happens on a local level. The Dutch police, for instance, work in several areas and in different projects using spyware and sucking up data to predict crimes and take judicial action. For this purpose, they use the system iColumbo, named after the apparently absent-minded detective with his worn-out trench coat from the TV series; the system automatically collects data from internet sites and analyses it with the aim of tracking crime. The police also hire commercial companies such as Coosto and HowAboutYou, that comb through the internet for suspicious activity and expressions on Facebook and Twitter. Using so-called sentiment analysis, the data is organised and analysed, so that people can be profiled based on positive, negative or neutrally labelled messages or given a risk profile.

One of the most famous examples of predictive policing is the Dutch police service's Criminaliteit Anticipatie Systeem (Criminality Anticipation System, CAS). Using a grid map of the Netherlands, with squares representing 125 metres by 125 metres, CAS indicates where and when there is the highest probability of 'high-impact crimes', such as street robberies and burglaries. They have set up an algorithm for this purpose which makes its way through a mountain of data taken from police reports and crime statistics, the police central data warehouse, and from public data such as the number of welfare payments per district to age, gender and family structures. This is done by establishing the risk of crime at various reference dates by means of an analysis of previous incidents in combination with the proximity of various risk factors, which can indicate that a particular neighbourhood in a particular city is at high risk of burglaries in the coming weeks. In this way, so-called 'heat maps' can be drawn up, indicating hotspots where the chance of certain forms of crime are highest. According to the Dutch police, 40% of burglaries and 60% of street robberies can be predicted this way.[2] It may even eventually be possible for the prediction to lead to a profile of a person indicating that they will be a criminal or victim in the future. This happens for instance in the heat map used by the Chicago police.[3]

The prediction police

The term 'predictive policing' became famous worldwide in 2008, when police commissioner William Bratton of the Los Angeles Police Department (LAPD) spoke at a public meeting in Los Angeles of the success of the police in tackling crime. Through predictive policing, according to Bratton's message, crime in the city had been significantly reduced. In particular the number of high-impact crimes, including assaults and gang violence in the city, had decreased substantially. Key to this is the software package PredPol (Predictive Policing), with which the LAPD predicts where and when crime will occur based on historical crime data. Jeffrey Brantingham, one of the co-founders of PredPol, describes predictive policing as a process that makes use of data to calculate the chance of future crime; the accuracy of the predictions is evaluated and the police are willing to intervene on the basis of the predictive information. In order to better tackle crime, other American police forces have begun to use PredPol. A year after Bratton's talk, Kristina Rose, acting director of the National Institute of Justice, acknowledged Police Commissioner Bratton as having 'served as the catalyst for bringing predictive policing to the forefront of police work'. It is expected that within a few years, every police force in American cities of 100,000 or more residents will make use of predictive policing.[4]

Besides PredPol, there are now predictive systems with names such as HunchLab (Philadelphia), Palantir (New Orleans), Precobs (Germany), ProMap (UK), KeyCrime (Italy), Maprevelation (France) and CAS (the Netherlands). What makes predictive policing so attractive to investigative agencies? How do they predict whether something will happen? Looking back is easier, is it not? The idea behind predictive policing is that predictions can be made about crimes on various levels. The first level of prediction is the location *where* particular crimes are committed and *what* those crimes are. The second level is about the point in time *when* something happens. Following from that, it might be possible to predict *who* would commit a crime. Finally, predictive policing makes it possible to combine where, what, when and who. All this is possible because crime is predictable to some extent, for instance because criminals often commit the same types of crimes. They also do so around the same locations, close to good escape routes and at the same times, often also with a relatively clear culprit profile. House break-ins or shop raids are familiar examples. Smart statistical methods make it possible to accelerate recognition of fixed or unusual patterns in types of behaviour that are exhibited relatively frequently, from speeding offences to credit card fraud.

In this new way of policing, the whole population is the battlefield.[5] Fixed or unusual patters in human behaviour are identified by analyses of large-scale data collections, including police data, and public sources that are tapped by learning algorithms. There is ever more data available to tell us about human behaviour, and there are also things around us that produce data (such as the internet of things). This is because we're constantly generating data, and all that data has predictive value. According to the latest figures, billions of people use WhatsApp every day, and Facebook is used every month by two billion people. The messages and conversations on these social media platforms can provide usable information about potential offenders. The results allow those using predictive policing to react faster to new incidents and focus their capacity based on the analyses. A trend indicating a substantial increase in the number of robberies in a particular part of Amsterdam leads to the police investing more in staffing and working hours in that part of the city.

Addicted to control

Predictive policing is a consequence of the control society we have ended up in. At the beginning of the 1990s, Gilles Deleuze wrote a brief – less than five pages – but influential article with the title *Post-scriptum sur les sociétés de contrôle* (Postscript on the Societies of Control).[6] His argument is that we live in a society in which everything revolves around control, a term which Deleuze borrows from a 'dour punk in a sharp suit', as NME's Leonie Cooper called the American novelist William S. Burroughs. In an interview with *Penthouse* in 1972, Burroughs argues that 'the means of control are much more efficient now. We have computers. [...] So the opportunities to control are much more potent now than they have ever been.' The control society according to Deleuze is the successor of what Michel Foucault describes as the disciplinary society, in which order is achieved within the limits of closed institutions, in prison, at school and in the factory. Deleuze notes that we are now experiencing an unprecedented technological revolution, and that with the arrival of new technologies, control has become a permanent process. It has become detached from the isolation of institutional environments and shifted into everyday life.

The ever greater scale on which control takes place is difficult to over-estimate. Driven by fear of terrorist attacks, crime and disorder, whether that fear is well-founded or not, a rampant need for control has taken over. This desire is expressed increasingly in camera surveillance, facial recognition systems, expanding police authorities, zero tolerance, preventative searches, area bans, drones, sensors, big data and gate systems that make it possible to deny people entry to locations such as metro and train stations. Not to mention an ever greater number of 'light blue' enforcers who are supposed to protect us: city supervisors, neighbourhood watch groups and private security services. The greed with which all this is deployed betrays a trend which has long been in motion and in which we attempt to avoid any form of misfortune at all costs. Criminologist Lucia Zedner speaks of a 'pre-crime-approach', where people no longer punish an infringement of the law, but seek to prevent potentially risky behaviour.[7]

A secure and certain future seems like a noble aim. Who can be against investigating crime? There is no experience as traumatic as insecurity, Freud would have said. Nevertheless, the need for ever stronger control seems contradictory in a time when crime figures in all Western countries continue to fall and the number of people feeling unsafe continues to drop. Not only are there fewer crimes and suspects, the number of criminal cases, sentences and prisoners is also now substantially lower. Figures from Statistics Netherlands (CBS) show that since 2002, crimes registered in the Netherlands have dropped by more than a quarter, and that the reduction applies to almost all crimes, from offences against property such as theft, burglary and muggings to violent crimes, traffic offences and vandalism. No wonder, then, that the prisons are empty. The number of people in prison in the Netherlands on an average day has dropped since 2005 from 14,000 to 9000. You can endlessly debate the issue of whether these figures are correct, but in fact they are quite consistent in their results. Both recorded crime (crime drop) and the number of people who sometimes feel insecure (fear drop) continue to fall. Add to that the fact that the number of people who say they have been victims of crime and the fact that in almost all Western countries the same drop in crime is taking place, and you have a clear picture. In times of hysteria it may seem a strange conclusion, but we live in a very safe part of the world. That makes it all the more relevant to ask why we're so fixated on insecurity in a society that has never been so safe. Where does the security hysteria come from?

Deleuze's article is too simple and insufficiently worked out to help us better understand why we still feel compelled to invest ever more in control. The image Deleuze sketches of the transition from a disciplinary to a control society is an appealing one, but it offers no answer to the question of why we want to be monitored in a society that is already very secure. Why do we long for our own monitoring?[8] In other words, what does our obsession with control over the society we live in say about us? An interesting starting point in answering this question is offered by William S. Burroughs in the character of the 'control addict', someone who is both addicted to control and obsessed by it; a character like Lacie Pound from *Black Mirror*. In an interview about his work in Ted Morgan's biography *Literary Outlaw*, Burroughs compares control with his lifelong drug addiction:

> The theory of addiction came into my head when the junk went into my arm. It was a metaphor for society. Addiction means somethin' that you've gotta have or you're sick. Power and junk are symmetrical and quantitative: How much?[9]

In the same interview, Burroughs points out that control primarily takes place in our heads and not through external force. Instead of someone else controlling us, we have come to internalise the control. We enthusiastically get to work on it, as if we were the police ourselves. This process goes so far, Burroughs feels, that it has led to a self-policing society. 'A functioning police state needs no police,' writes Burroughs in one of the most hallucinatory passages from his 1959 book *Naked Lunch*. Philosophically put, technological developments that promise to expand human freedom end up turning against that freedom, because they also increase our need for control.

Tell me your score, and I'll tell you who you are

We live in a culture of likes and smileys, where we are constantly exposing ourselves to everyone and at the same time watching others. Every day we can be found on Facebook, Instagram, Twitter and LinkedIn, sharing the most intimate details of our lives with others. Unasked and unabashed, we effectively make our entire lives transparent through WhatsApp, Facebook, Instagram and Twitter, knowing full well that most of the information is visible to everyone. You might call this behaviour hysterical. No one needs to be on their phone two hours a day looking at Facebook and Instagram for practical purposes. Many people have lost their grip on the time they spend on liking and sharing. They have lost control of their social media use and panic when they have no internet for a day. Online-neurosis is the term for this hysterical behaviour. At the same time, social media behaviour revolves around the look-at-me attitude, which the American social historian Christopher Lasch brilliantly called 'the culture of narcissism', that is part of the state of agitation in which we present and market ourselves. But what does it mean sociologically and culturally that we make the most personal confessions on a daily basis through the keyboard and on the screen? Why do we give ourselves over to total surveillance?

The book *Exposed* by American lawyer Bernard Harcourt offers an interesting starting point in more precisely delineating our behaviour on social media.[10] Harcourt speaks of our obsession with watching and being watched in terms of a power relationship that exploits our longing for visibility and strives for complete transparency. All this happens without the coercive elements of a disciplinary power. We are actively entranced – not passively. He calls this new power relationship 'expository power', and how this works becomes clear on the digital platforms of Apple, Netflix, Facebook and YouTube. These are intermediary channels where supply and demand meet. What is special about these platforms is that they have integrated and screened off the model of the network society, that is, the network itself. Content on such a platform can only be viewed when you're logged in, enabling monitoring of users' personal preferences such as interests, surfing habits and search terms, and making it clear how and when a person can be most effectively approached. If you often search for hotel discounts, there's a good chance you will begin to see ads for Booking.com on the websites you view.[11]

Although there are several ways that digital platforms deal with users and their data, they share the characteristic that you can acquire virtual credits – 'likes' on Facebook, 'views' on YouTube, 'followers' on Twitter or 'endorsements' on LinkedIn. Active users of these digital platforms expose themselves through videos, messages or photos in order to reach a broader public. Reaching an audience can have a professional goal, 'going viral' on YouTube for instance, in the case of vloggers promoting products and generating income from advertisers. But transparency can also serve a less concrete goal, such as a good feeling – a kick – when we're liked or retweeted. Research shows that the chemical dopamine, also known as the happy hormone, is released in our brains when we are successful on social media. Getting lots of likes on our Facebook page activates the reward circuit in our brain, while on the other hand, uncertainty strikes when we are unfollowed on Twitter or Facebook. It works in precisely the same way as drugs and other intoxicating substances, although the effects are not as strong.

All those likes and smileys also have a flipside. The grim 2018 documentary *The Cleaners* shows that Facebook intentionally elicits intense emotions in its users. Facebook's business model is focused on offering a platform to frustration and anger, emotions that are infectious and in combination with uncertainty often lead to hysteria. The more hysterical your post, the more clicks and views you generate and the greater the advertising revenue for Facebook. Like other social media, Facebook is built to encourage extreme messages and images by packaging them in short headlines and showing them in your timeline. It tries to maintain the user's attention for as long as possible. When such videos keep on cropping up in your timeline, it becomes more and more difficult to get out. Facebook is increasingly viewed as addictive, and with good reason.

Another phenomenon that feeds our desire for visibility and transparency is consumer scores that form the basis for financial advantages. As part of the terms of use of digital platforms, many companies allocate points to users. This has grown into a multi-billion-dollar industry, with Amazon, Google and Facebook emerging as the big earners, monetising the information you give away on digital platforms by selling them to companies that are interested in personalised marketing or who want to use the data to promote their own products or services. Although these kinds of ranking are as old as human civilisation, scoring through automated systems has expanded to all facets of life. Everyone receives a grade. Our own governments are also making frantic use of this, in every arena and without our knowledge. There are now truancy scores, health scores, threat scores, fraud scores, risk scores and so on ad infinitum. The scores determine whether you come under additional government scrutiny, but also allow you to get a loan or insurance. Detailed data on the behaviour of citizens and consumers determines whether you will be able to make use of a particular right or service in the future and at what price. Personal information is a currency – or in the terminology of the French anthropologist Marcel Mauss: a gift – in a kind of barter system. Although you might expect gift giving to have declined in late modernity, due to the increasingly impersonal nature of relationships, the advanced division of labour and a significant commercial sector, gift exchange remains a significant element in our society. Instead of physical objects such as tools, talismans, emblems, and food, reciprocity takes the form of handing over personal data or giving other parties access to monitor your data.[12] Financial advantages are then allotted to people who behave according to a particular lifestyle or positive behavioural norm. Car insurers, for instance, record your driving (speed, petrol consumption, etc.) with an app or device installed in your car. Based on your driving, they then keep a personal score. If you have a 'safe driving style', you receive a discount on your insurance premium: 35% for a safe driver and 10% for a reasonably safe driver. As a consequence, neither 'punishment and pleasure' nor 'commerce and surveillance' (data mining, profiling, monitoring) can be separated anymore.

What is important here is that the market power of the three-headed monster – Facebook, Amazon and Google – is paired with unprecedented data power. Google has access to a broad portfolio of products and services, from

Google Maps to YouTube and from Gmail to Android, used by billions of people worldwide. Everyone shops with Amazon, and Facebook connects everything and everyone. Market power and data power form a dangerous combination, certainly when the new Leviathan suffers from an insatiable hunger for data. It is only a matter of time before an algorithm comes along to combine all of a person's scores, bringing the 'dividual' from various media together to form a single 'in-dividual'. Facebook founder Mark Zuckerberg had something similar in mind with his dream of a universal social graph, a graphic map of all people's relationships and everything that interests them. At the annual Facebook conference F8 in May 2007, Zuckerberg told everyone present:

> The social graph is changing the way the world works. We are at a time in history when more information is available and people are more connected than they ever have been before, and the social graph is at the center of that.[13]

At F8 ten years on, Zuckerberg announced that the company was working on a brain scanner to read users' minds, using sensors connected to the part of the brain that deals with speech. In this way users would be able to communicate through thoughts, without having to physically engage with a device. For now, it is all a long way off and it remains unclear how all this would work, but Zuckerberg's dream is exactly the same as that of the intelligence services and the police.

'Holy shit, it's RoboCop'

These days people are not just citizens with rights and responsibilities, but also data streams to be tapped and analysed. Widespread surveillance and data collection maps out every detail of our lives, creating a world that previously only existed in gloomy science fiction films. The film world, like literature, has always been fascinated by high-tech weaponry and totalitarian regimes, as evidenced by works such as *Strange Days* by Kathryn Bigelow (1995), *The End of Violence* by Wim Wenders (1997), *Equilibrium* (2002) by Kurt Wimmer, *A Scanner Darkly* by Richard Linklater (2006) and *V for Vendetta* (2005) by James McTeigue. *Equilibrium* plays out in the authoritarian city state of Libria, a post-Third World War society led by the character Father. In order to avoid a new war, experiencing emotions and exercising free will are prohibited. So-called 'sense offenders', guilty of experiencing emotions and passions, are tracked down and eliminated by the police service *Grammaton Clerics*.

In *V for Vendetta*, based on the Alan Moore and David Lloyd's 1980s graphic novel by the same name, the UK is governed by the fascist Norsefire Party, which is systematically eradicating homosexuals, ethnic minorities and other 'deviants' from society. The main character, V, is a masked anarchist, modelled on Guy Fawkes, who attempted to topple King James I in the 17th century.

In the introduction to the graphic novel, Alan Moore explains that the story is a commentary on the England of the 1980s, when the Conservative prime minister Margaret Thatcher was in power for three terms:

> My youngest daughter is seven and the tabloid press are circulating the idea of concentration camps for persons with AIDS. The new riot police wear black visors, as do their horses, and their vans have rotating video cameras mounted on top. The government has expressed a desire to eradicate homosexuality, even as an abstract concept [...] I'm thinking of taking my family and getting out of this country soon.

There's sufficient reason to watch films that link the present with a future that looks even worse. I will focus on two films that are relevant to the theme of this chapter and which represent the extremes of the spectrum when it comes to police security enforcement: *RoboCop* (1987) by Paul Verhoeven and *Minority Report* (2002) by Steven Spielberg. The latter movie predicts a kind of law enforcement that operates like a smooth, super-efficient machine, while *Robocop* shows a far more gritty and extremely violent reality.

RoboCop is set in the year 2029. Utter chaos reigns in Detroit. Countless attacks and other violent crimes are committed on a daily basis. During a chase, police officer Alex Murphy is peppered with bullets by a gang of criminals. First his right hand is shot to pieces, then they shoot his arm off, and on top of that he takes a bullet to the head. Murphy perches on the brink of death, but the Security Concepts department at Omni Consumer Products ('OmniCorp') succeeds in keeping him alive and making him into a police officer who is half human, half machine. His programmers have set three rules that he must comply with (1) 'serve the public trust', (2) 'protect the innocent' and (3) 'uphold the law'. Multinational OmniCorp specialises in robot technologies. Their robots are used to wage war on behalf of the United States all over the world, and now the company wants to deploy its products in the big cities of the US that are plagued with crime. Using digital implants and technological applications in Murphy's head and upper body, OmniCorp ensures that he can simply continue with his work. This goes beyond the distinction between 'good cop' and 'bad cop', to paraphrase Friedrich Nietzsche, hence the name, 'RoboCop'. It is something between man and machine, an electronic Frankenstein: 'Part Man, Part Machine, All Cop'.

RoboCop is about the effect of the fusion of man and machine, biology and technology, on fighting crime. The film raises a number of salient issues, such as how the Irish Catholic Alex Murphy is turned into an ideal fighting machine, invincible to bullet and bombs and equipped with high-tech weaponry. The idea being that Murphy's human brain should keep the robot inside under control, he is Terminator and Rambo in one; the only human part of him visible to the public is the lower part of his face. His equipment makes him superior in every respect to the classic police officer. Not only is he stronger and faster, he also has the most sophisticated military weapons to take down criminals.

The hypermilitarisation of the police which *RoboCop* depicts is not just an American phenomenon; it is also increasingly visible in other countries. When batons and pepper spray prove ineffective, many European police forces currently use tasers, weapons which deliver a brief electric current, causing the muscles to contract so that a person loses control of their body. Arming the police increasingly heavily is part of a worldwide trend in an attempt to win back their lost authority on the street. Watching *RoboCop*, it is difficult not to be constantly thinking of what the American writer Ta-Nehisi Coates called the 'Gospel of Giuliani', after the former mayor of New York who constantly harped on about more 'law and order'. At the same time, we see that the hypermilitarisation of the police goes further than the arming of officers alone – the politics of 'law and order' also makes use of metaphors and images derived from the army, such as 'war on crime' and 'war on drugs', which were discussed in detail in Chapter 3. In his book *Rise of the Warrior Cop*, American journalist Radley Balko outlines the gradual evolution of the militarisation of police forces. In the conclusion of his book, he writes: 'Police today are armed, dressed, trained, and conditioned like soldiers.'[14]

While RoboCop, resurrected in steel, deploys a zero tolerance policy in the violent streets of Detroit, the film *Minority Report* presents a very different view of the police. In Washington DC in the year 2054, there is no fighting force armed to the teeth; instead, there is a police appliance at work behind the scenes to predict who will commit a crime. The film is based on a short story by Philip K. Dick, published in 1956 in the magazine *Fantastic Universe*. In contrast to the work of many of his fellow-writers in the 1950s and 1960s, his stories are characterised by a pessimistic tone and a deep mistrust of the authorities. Among the wider public, Dick was famous for the film *Blade Runner* by director Ridley Scott, a film adaptation of his 1968 story *Do Androids Dream of Electric Sheep?* But definitive recognition of Dick as a writer of visionary stories came in 2002 with the film *Minority Report*, in which Tom Cruise plays a police captain on the run, attempting to avoid a murder that he himself is predicted to commit. Three years before Spielberg started work on the production of *Minority Report*, he invited 16 specialists, including William Mitchell (author of *City of Bits*), writer Douglas Coupland, computer scientist Neil Gershenfeld and urban designer Peter Calthorpe, to consider the future of the city and the management of crime and disorder. They came up with three paranormal 'pre-cogs', connected by a 'hive mind', a group consciousness, capable of predicting future murders.

References to *Minority Report* are gradually becoming the norm when it comes to the terrifying spectre of a future in which privacy is non-existent and the police creep into the heads of citizens. Nevertheless, the film is too valuable to dismiss as a cliché. What is particularly interesting is the way it reveals how the constitutional quality of crime prevention is safeguarded. Based on the precogs' predictions, the names of victim and culprit and the time of the crime are engraved in wooden balls. Then a special procedure is followed consisting of various precisely defined protocols, the most important of which involves the head of the Pre-Crime Unit, police commissioner John Anderton, reading out the name of the victim and the culprit in the presence of two witnesses, Dr Katherine James and Chief Justice Frank Pollard. While the entire procedure is filmed, James and Pollard check whether the names read out match those engraved in the two balls. They grant their approval, then the agents from the Pre-Crime Unit set off right away for the scene of the crime to arrest the 'culprit' before the crime can be committed. That person is then imprisoned without trial. 'In our society we have no major crimes', John Anderton says. 'We have a detention camp full of would-be-criminals.'

Computer says yes

In fact, it is surprising how conservative futuristic films such as *RoboCop* and *Minority Report* are in their estimation of technological developments in our society – Verhoeven and Spielberg were also influenced by the views of their time. Although *Minority Report* is set in 2054, a police force that tracks people down before they commit crimes is not as far away as it appears at face value. Yesterday's future has already caught up with us. What was science fiction in *Minority Report* is reality today, as Police Commissioner William Bratton stated a couple of years ago in a debate about big data and security. That this is not just about the predictive and algorithmic models of police computers, is shown in the Netherlands, where the National Police uses psychics when investigating serious crimes. Former Minister of Justice Ivo Opstelten justified the use of these living oracles under the following circumstances: 'There has to be a serious crime involved, and the investigation must have reached a dead end using the usual research methods.'

Predictive police work is an attractive idea, and one that appeals to the imagination of many a politician and policy maker. Advocates of this policy believe that predictive policing is the next step in technological developments that will substantially improve police work. Through analysis of large quantities of data, more crimes are more precisely predicted, allowing the police to intervene faster and in a more targeted way to the threat of crime, for instance by providing surveillance in the right place. The approach can reveal blind spots in tracking, relating to crimes of which the police have insufficient knowledge or none at all, and the overstretched police force can deploy its scarce resources more efficiently. Predictive policing is not only seen as positive from the perspective of combating crime, but could also be a tool for improving the protection of citizens. Prejudice and discrimination would have less of a chance, because an impersonal algorithm would be used: the judgement of a computer is rather more objective than that of the average police officer.

Nevertheless, the effect of this digital crystal ball raises various issues. How does the flipside of this solution look? What are the dark sides of this new dataism? For a start, making correct predictions as to who will toe the line and who will not is highly dependent on the quality of the data to which the predictive policing algorithm has access. While in principle the word 'data' covers everything as long as it is digital, in practice, not all data will be equally useful. Data experts argue that 'dirty data' in police practices, created from flawed, racially biased, and unlawful practices, cause discriminatory results, leading to over-policing of high-poverty and non-white urban areas. Critical scholars speak of 'the New Jim Code' to refer to how data reproduce existing inequities in society.[15]

Predictive policing works on the basis of historical facts, such as the number of burglaries or robberies in a city. This means that the system does not so much predict as extrapolate the chance of something happening – it analyses crime from the past, not that of the future. 'Predicting the present' would actually be a better way of describing what these systems do. The danger in all this is that a self-reinforcing effect arises in police work; it becomes a self-fulfilling prophecy. If the police more frequently keep watch on deprived areas of London, more police data will be collected from these neighbourhoods, so that the predictive policing algorithms will be more likely to highlight these areas as hotspots. This self-reinforcing effect will become stronger and stronger because not all crime appears in police statistics, as not all crimes are reported to or discovered by the police; this is termed the 'dark figure of crime'. Precise figures are hard to come by, but it is estimated that more than 70% of all crime is not reported to the police. This means that the police mainly focus on crime that is already known. A white businessman committing fraud on the London Stock Exchange will not be seen in the digital crystal ball of predictive policing because the police pay less attention to financial crime, certainly compared with issues such as theft, murder and rape.

Correct predictions of crime are also difficult to make because the algorithms and data used are never neutral. An algorithm, for instance, is not an objective calculating aid without character or direction. It is set up by developers, analysts and policy makers, which in many cases makes it politically sensitive. To put it technically, this entails that there is always a bias in the software used to predict crime, which can ultimately lead to discrimination. Often the users of the software have no way of finding out why the system has come to a particular decision, as exerting control on the opaque algorithm is almost completely impossible. This problem became most apparent in a 2016 investigation into the risk profiles of the American justice system by the journalist platform Pro-Publica. More and more US judges use the algorithms of the company Northpointe to calculate the chance of a suspect committing more crimes in the future, and base their verdict on the outcome. If the chance of recidivism is higher, then a more severe prison sentence is imposed. The investigation by ProPublica into this form of predictive justice shows that the algorithm sends people with a darker skin colour to prison for longer. Convicts with darker skin are systematically allocated higher risk scores than white convicts. Thus dark-skinned people wrongly emerge from the risk systems as future criminals twice as often as white people, regardless of whether they have previously been convicted of an offence. ProPublica's conclusion is that the algorithm used works little better than tossing a coin.

Finally, the privacy of citizens will always be the subject of discussion. With predictive policing, the chance of privacy being infringed is high because the algorithms were not thought up or developed with privacy in mind. Furthermore, as much information as possible is processed and as many datasets as possible are linked in order to identify correlations and patterns of crime by citizens. This easily leads to action in conflict with the legal principle of purpose limitation, which states that information can only be used and processed for a defined, clearly delimited and justified goal. Predictive policing is further at odds with the principle of necessity, which entails that the data collection should be limited to the strictly necessary, because the data of innocent citizens is also involved. All in all, predictive policing in its ideal form would involve the collection of as much data as possible ('bigger is better'), including data that was originally intended for goals other than investigating crime. To a certain extent, therefore, the infringement of privacy is part and parcel of predictive policing.

Surveillance continuum

'PreCrime, it works!', states the slogan of John Anderton's police unit in *Minority Report*. The promise of predictive policing is that we can have a carefree existence, that everything is controllable and predictable, far from the hysteria linked with the remaining bit of insecurity in our society. The question is then how that use of data, algorithms and statistics relates to the way the classic police officer works. How does it fundamentally alter ordinary forms of policing and governance? The police's new modus operandi is, after all, diametrically opposed to approaches based on investigating a crime that has taken place and imposing punishments reactively – now, the police want to intervene before a crime has even taken place. The correlations and patterns (descriptive) which make it possible to predict people's behaviour and actions (predictive) direct the police in their investigative activities (prescriptive) to arrest suspects ahead of time.

In what I will refer to as a 'surveillance continuum', predictive policing leads to a series of other tracking activities with the aim of actively steering the future. This means that predictive policing is not an isolated phenomenon, but is always linked to other police methods. The two most important methods in this situation are 'hotspot policing' and 'ethnic profiling'. Hotspot policing is targeted, long-term tackling of particular spots in a neighbourhood where a great deal of crime takes place, for instance in an apartment block, a park or a town square with pavement cafés. The idea behind this is that work should continue on making these hotspots safe until it is no longer seen as a problem area. According to Franklin Zimring, this form of intervention has proven successful in tackling crime in New York.[16] An important force behind this is the introduction of the crime database CompStat ('Computer Stats') into the working processes of the New York City Police Department (NYPD). CompStat is a statistical program which provides real-time crime information by making smart use of all information that could be relevant in combating crime.

The advantage of CompStat is that the NYPD gains faster, more accurate information about crime in the various neighbourhoods of New York. For instance, with this system hotspots can be identified that were not previously known to the police. Zimring, however, also points out that in practice the hotspot approach is mainly applied in deprived areas of the city and in places where a lot of people from ethnic minorities live. In this way, the method reinforces the unfair relationships between different groups. The hotspots approach also goes hand in hand with invasive and aggressive policing methods, including the 'Stop-and-Frisk' programme (a form of preventive searching), whereby people can be stopped at random and searched on suspicion of criminal activity. This method is very controversial, because experience shows that people of ethnic minorities are stopped far more frequently than white people. While as much as 85% of the almost van 4.5 million searches in New York between 2004 and 2012 involved black or Latino men, in only 6% of cases did this lead to arrest. Stop-and-Frisk has since been judged unconstitutional by a federal judge; in the case of *Floyd v. City* of New York in 2013, Judge Shira Scheindlin reached the verdict that Stop-and-Frisk violated articles of the Constitution that prohibit unreasonable detention and guarantee equal treatment.

In this way, security hysteria can become an ugly obstruction to justice, particularly when methods such as predictive policing lead to profiling on the basis of ethnicity: a form of policing that is socially unacceptable, because it mainly affects minorities. In ethnic profiling, people are more frequently checked by the police based on their ethnic background, even when they have committed no offence. This means that citizens are disproportionately frequently detained by the police based on their ethnic background or skin colour, without an objective or reasonable justification. According to Amnesty International, this kind of 'gut feeling check' happens systematically in many countries, while the practice is out of proportion with the level of individual incidents, the human rights organisation claims. Other research also shows that the police intervene selectively against people with immigrant backgrounds based on external characteristics. Besides non-white skin colour, factors such as age, gender and particular clothing styles also play a role. For instance, the much-used Dutch police term 'target group' is mainly used to refer to youths with a Moroccan background.[17] Recently, the directors of various police forces have drawn up a code of conduct to prevent police officers from applying ethnic profiling. In spite of that, it is an open secret that many officers consider such profiling completely normal, convinced as they are that more criminals are caught this way. That is not supported by the facts, however; in practice, it turns out that officers substantially overestimate the effectiveness of their own intuition. The police officer's gut feeling is almost always completely wrong.[18]

Digital police trap

It is mainly the success stories of predictive policing that have become famous, and that is not completely unwarranted. Predictive policing seems fruitful when it comes to predicting the locations where relatively simple crimes such as burglaries and street robberies will take place. Predicting who will commit offences and when they will happen, however, is rather more difficult, particularly when it comes to complicated crimes such as terrorism; the problem is that risk profiles are far too broad to make precise predictions as to the people who will commit an attack and the time when they will do it. Not only does the information used for the analyses become dated, the process also spits out many more suspects than the security services can keep watch on. Moreover, the advocates of predictive policing forget that the average terrorist knows perfectly well that everyone is permanently under surveillance. Coded language and encrypted messages online are therefore ever on the rise.

But there are more issues with the digital police trap. With the shift from a post-crime to a pre-crime approach, the aim and reach of the investigation of criminal offences also changes radically. Predictive policing, after all, takes place on the border between suspicion and conduct, because it involves taking an advance on what a person is going to do in the future. It is a speculative security discourse that anticipates the question: 'What might happen?' A risk of this penal divination is that in estimating the risk of someone exhibiting criminal behaviour, you also increase the tendency to place people's state of mind or inner disposition under suspicion, in the absence of a concrete criminal offence. Individuals could be sentenced based on statistically probable behaviour instead of what they have actually done. In connection with this, we might point to the expansion of penal provisions around terrorism in the penal code, so that what applies to intentions becomes directly relevant to the question of whether the suspect is preparing an act of terrorism. I would like to dwell a bit longer on this rarely discussed but important effect of predictive policing in order to better understand the shady side of security hysteria.

In penal law, the criminal act (i.e. the actual offence committed) has always been central. Criminal responsibility applies exclusively to the criminal act. This is known as the *nulla poena sine lege poenali* principle: there can be no punishment without an act that is prohibited by law. The term 'act' here assumes a specific decision on the part of a person. This perspective is based on a physical or causal theory of action, better known as the 'voluntary muscle movement'. In this respect an act is only criminally relevant if the cause of the muscle movement is intentional. In other words, a criminal act must be expressed or made externally visible by means of a specific decision on the part of a person. The notion of a voluntary muscle movement has since been replaced by a more functional notion of committing a crime. The question now is, what is perceived as an action under existing standards, rules and practices. Nevertheless, it remains the case that penal law is not concerned purely with the inner lives of citizens. Thoughts are free. This goes back, among other origins, to the principle in Roman law of *cogitationis poenam nemo patitur*, which amounts to the idea that no one can be exposed to punishment for thoughts alone.

There are various arguments to be made as to why penal law in general and the police in particular should not concern themselves with people's thoughts. After all, having thoughts about a crime does not have to lead to actually committing the offence. Someone wanting to commit a terrorist attack may repent in time. By focusing on thoughts, the prediction police also read too much into behaviour that is not particularly significant in itself. The police look into the heads of citizens by giving meaning to intentions that are generally difficult to pin down, thus placing themselves in the psychiatrist's chair. In 2015, for instance, the Dutch court acquitted a suspect of preparing a terrorist attack due to insufficient evidence. When it came to trial, the file and the investigation showed that the suspect had merely possessed a notebook in which he had written down a recipe for an explosive, among other things, and that he had presented himself in chats on Facebook as a supporter of Islamic State.

All this can lead to a random and even more premature deployment of tracking methods and technology by the police, without oversight from a judge. Predictive policing, after all, uses a tracking method against non-suspects in the hope of unearthing a random crime. In the absence of concrete suspicion, large quantities of personal data are collected with a view to future offences. Investigations expand in this way to include people who are not yet under suspicion and without their knowledge. This leads to an area ungoverned by law, one in which the norm and deviation are indistinguishable, but where it is necessary to make a decision as to the distinction. In this space, the decision-making power shifts from the judiciary to executive authorities such as the police.

Taking into account the shift from post-crime to pre-crime, in the context of this chapter it can be stated that the possible applications of predictive policing threaten to take us ever further from classic penal law, whereby a person's action is central. Very large quantities of data, such as giving out likes in response to Facebook and Twitter messages, which in turn come from different sources, lead to the extrapolation of the possible realisation of a criminal consequence. At the same time, it is unclear which indications are required before the prediction police intervene, as decisions on this are no longer made via a clear chain of command. They are also no longer stated on paper, but are included in the software of search engines of algorithmic police and intelligence services. Since we run the risk of losing sight of the criminally relevant action, the threshold for criminality will shift towards intention; the presumed intention will become more important than concrete action – *Gesinnungsstrafrecht*, as it is termed in German, referring to the fact that a belief that was considered wrong and not to be tolerated constituted a criminal offence under Adolf Hitler's National Socialist regime. Is it sufficient evidence to convict someone if he or she regularly visits a mosque, makes use of the website justpaste.it, which is popular among ISIS supporters, and books a flight to the Middle East? What interpretation should we give to these non-criminal offences? In short, who still dares to be themselves?

Conclusion

Hysteria is infectious, and social media such as Facebook, Twitter and Instagram cause it to spread faster. It is an emotional or collective infection without contact between people, in which intense emotional states transferred via real-life social networks can lead to large-scale infections. This in turn has an effect on behaviour in the real world, especially when people regard shocking events as the end of the world. Facebook and YouTube have made this their business model, with recommendation algorithms ensuring that hysterical messages and extreme images gain priority in your timeline. This keeps us glued to our screens for longer and we become afraid of missing something, the uncomfortable feeling that others are having all kinds of rewarding experiences in our absence. But it is not only Facebook and YouTube that make smart use of our need to share everything – the police have also discovered that the messages and conversations on social media provide useful information for predicting crime. Predictive policing, where the police operate as a kind of thought police and arrest you even before you have done anything, is proof of this.

Faith in algorithms as predictors of truth in tracking and trying suspects is visibly – almost hysterically – on the increase. Hysteria, however, often turns out to offer unwise counsel. If the benefits of predictive policing are real, then so are its risks. Mistakes lie in wait, because the predictions reflect prejudices in the data, and what is more, the principles of rule of law are at stake. There is a danger that detaining suspects faster and earlier constitutes a conflict with the principles of law, including the presumption of innocence. Additionally, predictive policing is not a method deployed in isolation; it forms part of a surveillance continuum that also involves hotspot policing and ethnic profiling. Ethnic minorities, in particular, are the victims of these police activities. Finally, predictive policing gives rise to the risk of penal consequences being imposed based on intentions that are difficult to pin down and actions which in themselves are insignificant, innocent everyday behaviour, such as buying a plane ticket to the Middle East or following a course about a particular religion.

Citizens have hardly any control over the use of algorithms by police and intelligence services. There is no transparency as to the choices made in implementing the algorithms in the predictive systems. We have no idea what is inside those black boxes that make decisions about us, even though that is our data, those are our lives. The algorithms of tech giants such as Facebook and Google, which personalise our internet experience and are used to sell us things, hardly seem threatening. When they sell opinions, however, they can corrupt democracy. But if the same algorithms and decision models determine the course of the criminal justice system, they have the potential to do immense damage.

All this impels us to reflect. We have long thought that a pleasant and secure society requires us to keep checks on one another. The government keeps check on citizens and citizens on the government. But the arrival of data-driven predictive systems turns everything on its head. The question now is: who keeps check on the algorithms?

Notes

1 Zuboff (2019).
2 Willems & Doeleman (2014).
3 Ferguson (2017).
4 There are two variants of predictive policing. The Dutch system, CAS, is a form of prediction known as *predictive mapping*, a temporal and spatial analysis focused on mapping out the 'when' and 'where' of a crime. *Predictive identification*, the second variant, goes a step further, indicating people or groups as potential criminals or victims. One of the most emotive applications of this is the Chicago police system, which indicates 'hot persons', who are expected to commit a crime in the near future. Other American cities use similar systems, including New Orleans, where the police work with the datamining company Palantir Technologies for this purpose.
5 Bernard Harcourt speaks in his compelling 2018 book *The Counterrevolution* of a 'counterinsurgency war paradigm' of which a fully transparent population is the first requisite.
6 Deleuze (1990, pp. 240–247).
7 Zedner (2007).
8 In this connection, it is interesting to note that after the fall of the Berlin Wall, citizens were allowed to inspect the vast archive of the Stasi, East Germany's secret service (the *Ministerium für Staatssicherheit* in full), and were disappointed when their names did not appear in the 111 kilometres of files belonging to the intelligence and security service. The most revealing point here is not the large scale on which citizens were monitored, but that they wanted to be monitored.
9 Morgan (2012, p. 351).
10 Harcourt (2015).
11 The practical implication of this is that there are more and more ads looking at us, instead of us looking at ads. The film *Minority Report* (2002) presents a fascinating picture of how customised advertising works. In a magnificent scene the main character John Anderton runs, agitated and hounded, through a warehouse while avatars on digital screens equipped with facial recognition software screen his face and call out his name to get his attention. The virtual shop assistants in the warehouse show him products fully tailored to his unique profile. 'John Anderton: you could use a Guinness right about now,' one avatar says. Fiction or reality? The first step in this direction has already been taken in train stations, at bus stops and in large shopping centres, where digital advertising pillars are equipped with cameras that monitor passers-by. They measure how many people are looking at a particular advert and how long for. They also observe whether a person is happy with the advert displayed.
12 Schuilenburg & Peeters (2017).
13 'Facebook Unveils Platform for Developers of Social Applications', 24 May 2007, retrieved from https://about.fb.com/news/2007/05/facebook-unveils-platform-for-developers-of-social-applications
14 Balko (2013, p. 333).
15 Benjamin (2019).
16 Zimring (2012).
17 Çankaya (2012).
18 Landman & Kleijer-Kool (2016, p. 183 ff.).

Chapter 6

So you think you can participate?

Introduction

Hysteria has always been with us, just like our constant need to fight it. No other condition has been treated in such a variety of ways, always with the aim of wiping it out for good. But it seems that the harder we try to stamp out hysteria, the more tenaciously it returns. As I have shown in Chapter 2, for example, the narrative of hysteria was dominated by devils and demons for centuries. Hysteria and the devil had been intrinsically linked since early Christendom, when the condition was assumed to be Satan's doing and usually manifested itself in individuals, though whole communities could sometimes be affected. At the time, the fight against hysteria, and the driving out of demons in particular, was a religiously charged affair – in the age of the Inquisition, hysteria was firmly a matter of exorcism. Preachers with close ties to God diagnosed people as hysterical and had them burnt at the stake.

In the course of the 18th century, new medical insights about hysteria won terrain, taking the condition out of the religious sphere and allowing prejudiced beliefs about the devil to give way to interest in the disease's neurological causes. Increasingly, hysteria was treated at hospitals and patients' behaviour monitored by physicians, most famously Jean-Martin Charcot, a neurologist at the Salpêtrière hospital in Paris. As Foucault would later say, the cure was a matter of normalisation. At the close of the 19th century, Freud severed this alleged link between hysteria and neurological illness, or more specifically, disorders of the brain. He considered hysteria a psychiatric phenomenon caused by suppressed memories and fantasies, often of a sexual nature, and his research into the condition gave him a better understanding of human sexuality. His most important method of treatment, perfectly in line with the psychological nature of hysteria, focused on bringing about mental changes in his patients. It was the beginning of what would later be called free association, a technique in which the patient tells the therapist everything that pops into their mind without censor.

Hysteria's transformation from a religious phenomenon to a medical model increasingly led to a new understanding and treatment of the condition, and as a result, many assumptions, ideas and treatment methods that have informed the history of hysteria are no longer valid today. But for proof that hysteria is still alive and kicking, you only need to look as far as the current sense of insecurity ordinary citizens feel in their immediate surroundings – and which they blame on others. Loitering youth, dogs, and immigrants have all made perfectly decent neighbourhoods 'uninhabitable'. Local residents label a bunch of annoying teenagers 'street terrorists', put up signs prohibiting barking dogs (the 'barking ban') and declare that newcomers to their neighbourhood are out to 'rape our daughters'. Hysteria being a contagious emotion, any discussion culminates in the same feverish cacophony. There seems to be no turning back from the slippery slope to the Apocalypse.

'Angry citizens' are symptomatic of these hysterical times, and in an attempt to assuage their violent reactions, the government is looking for new ways of getting a handle on hysteria. One of the most commonly used methods to achieve this is by involving local communities in initiatives to improve the liveability of their neighbourhoods, in the hope that giving residents more say will help them manage their rage and agitation. Recent years have seen many experiments based on this method, in which hysteria is turned into a govern-ance model, such as the Buurt Bestuurt (Neighbourhood Takes Charge) initiative in the Rotterdam Hillesluis neighbourhood, where local residents are consulted on how to tackle the biggest problems in their local area. What problems those are is decided by the residents of Hillesluis themselves. But just how seriously does the government take these Hillesluis activists? Does this initiative actually reduce hysteria and boost citizens' trust in the government? To answer this, I would like to give a brief introduction to a frustrated and angry Dutch neighbourhood.

A brief history

The Rotterdam neighbourhood of Hillesluis has a reputation as a stereotypical socially deprived area. Located in the district Feijenoord on the south side of Rotterdam, it is divided into North Rieder, South Rieder and the Walraven and Slaghek quarters. Like other neighbourhoods in South Rotterdam, Hillesluis was built at the beginning of the 19th century, at a time when there was a great demand for cheap labour in the port of Rotterdam. A typical working-class neighbourhood, it consists of narrow roads densely packed for the greater part with blocks of cheap, small flats of between 60 and 80 square metres in size. Half of them are council flats and only a quarter privately owned. The population originally consisted of dockworkers, mainly from the provinces Zeeland and North Brabant, but rapidly became more diverse after the Second World War, when indigenous Dutch residents were replaced by immigrant workers from Turkey and Morocco who squeezed into the cramped flats with their families. Today, the population of Hillesluis – once known colloquially as 'the farmers' quarter' because of its huge number of Dutch farmworkers – is largely composed of people with a predominantly Turkish background. A quarter of the 12,000 residents of Hillesluis are now of Turkish origin (25.1%), while the Dutch make up 20.9% of the neighbourhood, the Dutch Surinamese 13.9% and the Dutch Moroccans 10.2%. The other 30% is made up of citizens from dozens of other backgrounds.

Prominent landmarks of the neighbourhood are the Essalam Mosque, whose 2600 square metres make it the largest mosque of the Netherlands, and the South Shopping Boulevard that runs across Hillesluis in a straight line from Beijerland Lane and the Groene Hilledijk Street down to Sandeling Square. Over a kilometre in length and lined with more than 240 shops, the shopping street has the highest concentration of retailers in the sub-district Feijenoord, and was known as one of Rotterdam's most vibrant areas half a century ago. It had everything from a wide range of shops and restaurants to the Colosseum Cinema, but started to go downhill when the Zuidplein Mall opened its doors in the adjacent Charlois neighbourhood in the 1970s. The same year saw the first race riots of the Netherlands, which I will discuss in more detail in the next chapter. The rioting broke out nearby the shopping boulevard one warm summer evening in August, when a Dutch woman was evicted by her Turkish landlord, and despite the massive police action, it took a week for the turmoil to settle. In the years that followed, the range of shops changed dramatically, as the changing population of the neighbourhood brought with it the first Turkish butchers and greengrocers. Today, Turkish, Papiamento, Hindi and Arabic are spoken in the street, which, combined with the many kebab places and bridal shops, give the South Shopping Boulevard an atmosphere redolent of that of foreign cities. But various attempts to revive the high street have failed to improve its bad image, as dwindling visitor numbers, poor turnover, limited range of retailers, empty shops and high crime and offence levels show only too plainly. It has been nicknamed variously 'Whitewash Street', 'Headache Street' and 'Doner Kebab Street'.

In 2009, Hillesluis was named as one of the 40 most deprived neighbourhoods in the Netherlands, due to its residents' poor socio-economic circumstances. Seventy per cent of Hillesluis households lived on a low income, significantly more than the Rotterdam average of 51%. A mere 5% of residents earned a high income and 25% a middle income, compared with 16% and 33% respectively in the rest of the city. Many residents also struggle with poor literacy in Dutch and a low average level of education compared with other parts of Rotterdam. As a result, the neighbourhood has performed badly on the Social Development Index for years, its lowest score being 4.5 out of 10. The scarcity of social capital is exacerbated by the residents' lack of lobbying and organisational skills, and their distrust of government. The neighbourhood also knows a high turnover of residents – people tend not to stay long, with 21% of all homes inhabited for less than two years. Compared with other neighbourhoods, Hillesluis has a young population, with 30% of residents being under 18. It also has the lowest safety score of all Rotterdam neighbourhoods, and children are exposed to drugs, violence, burglaries and guns.

As a result of this situation, public trust in politics has reached an all-time low in Hillesluis. Weighed down by misery, crime and exclusion, residents no longer feel at home in their own neighbourhood. Many of them feel a kind of resigned despondency about their situation. Poverty? A given. Shootings? Come with the territory. Dealing drugs? Doesn't everyone. A situation like this can easily turn into frustration, anger and even hysteria, and it is why such feelings need to be taken seriously. Just like fear, which I have discussed in Chapter 3, frustration and anger are staple ingredients of hysteria, which makes it important to find out what exactly the residents of Hillesluis are angry about.

Neighbourhood Takes Charge

A lot has been written and said on the subject of hysteria among citizens, often without consulting the citizens themselves or asking what has caused their violent emotions. Why do so many people believe that their neighbourhood is in complete chaos? To find out, I spent some time hanging out in the Rotterdam neighbourhood of Hillesluis and joined the North Rieder Neighbourhood Takes Charge group for two years.[1]

Neighbourhood Takes Charge (NTC) is a fairly recent initiative aimed at improving liveability and strengthening social cohesion in Hillesluis. It was developed in 2009 by the Rotterdam police officer Hans Hoekman and head of the neighbourhood police team Fons Bijl, who believed that the gap between the police and the public had become too wide to adequately respond to problems faced by citizens. Inspired by other Dutch projects such as Veilige Buurten (Safe Neighbourhoods) in Maastricht, the two policemen devised a plan to form a residents' committee and launched a pilot of the NTC project in the Rotterdam Pupillen neighbourhood.

Other sources of inspiration were American projects such as the Chicago Alternative Police Strategy (CAPS). First developed in the mid-1990s, it allowed residents to set their own agenda to identify problems in the area, as well as giving them a say in how such issues should be tackled by the city council and police. Wesley Skogan's research into the results of the CAPS project show a marked increase in safety in deprived areas of Chicago, as well as a significant rise in public trust in politics.[2] Remarkably, this increase in trust was felt across various ethnic groups, ranging from African Americans to Latinxs. A similar approach taking place in Great Britain is called reassurance policing, in which police take action by focusing on so-called signal crimes and providing feedback of the results to the community. Evaluations have shown that this has also brought about a substantial increase in actual and perceived safety, as well as trust in the government.

An average NTC committee consists of between 10 and 15 members – though this number can be twice as large in some Rotterdam neighbourhoods – and a core team consisting of a local police officer, urban management officials and a council liaison officer. Other participants of NTC may include local community organisations such as DOCK, which is a foundation aiming to improve residents' ability to organise themselves and is also represented on the North Rieder committee. The main goal of NTC is to improve the neighbourhood's liveability. Besides increasing actual safety in the neighbourhood, the council aims to enhance the residents' sense of security – for as I showed in Chapter 4, when residents lose their trust in the government, their sense of security also deteriorates rapidly. The project also has the aim of enhancing mutual trust between residents and government by giving local communities a real say in how problems in their neighbourhoods should be addressed, as well as a number of unofficial – though no less important – goals such as improving residents' self-reliance and a more goal-oriented and effective use of public services. Finally, NTC is a tool for gauging what works and what does not work to improve the neighbourhood's liveability. It has shown, for instance, that citizens are often badly informed of the government's range of duties and the level of influence it has on certain problems.

NTC follows a very straightforward procedure: by suggesting ideas to improve liveability in their neighbourhood, residents have a direct influence on government policy and exercise their right to participation ('having a say'). They draw up a list of the three most pressing local problems that need to be solved, and the council and police get to work on tackling them while actively involving the residents in the process. In so-called short-term feedback, the government informs the residents of the results at the NTC meetings before the whole process begins again, in a continued effort to work towards higher liveability in the neighbourhood. The city council received the NTC method with great enthusiasm, and Mayor of Rotterdam Ahmed Aboutaleb announced in his New Year's speech that it would be introduced in all boroughs of the city as one of the spearheads of the Rotterdam security programme. The police and Rotterdam Urban Management allocated 200 extra hours of police presence per NTC branch to be used to address the problems raised by the residents.

Giving citizens a say

Citizen participation in government policy has long passed the experimental stage in the Netherlands, as local communities have firmly established themselves as an extension of the government. More and more citizens take an active part in carrying out duties in the public domain, and under the guise of 'hands-on democracy' the responsibility for and implementation of government policies is increasingly shared with the citizens. This shift from the state to non-state parties addressing government issues could be described as making government policies open to the public, a process that distinguishes between different forms of involvement and, by extension, of different groups of the public and their distinct identities. By 'groups of the public', I mean groups of individuals with shared experiences or a common interest, gathering for short or extended periods. It is difficult to give a comprehensive list, but they currently take the form of neighbourhood meetings, neighbourhood watch schemes, neighbourhood and residents' budget groups as well as citizens' councils and juries, public polls, neighbourhood development groups and participation groups. For citizens, much of the promise that the shift of responsibility from the state to the public holds is an increased freedom to determine how to run their own lives. To free people from the nanny state, you must give them more freedom to do things their own way.

The political philosopher Isaiah Berlin provided the basis for this idea with the twin terms 'positive liberty' and 'negative liberty'.[3] Negative liberty means not being hindered by obstacles or constraints ('freedom from'), while positive liberty means being given the opportunity to improve your life ('freedom to'). Negative liberty lies at the heart of classic liberalism, an interpretation of liberty that protects society against too much state intervention. Positive liberty is harder to define – at its core lies the freedom of citizens to develop and thrive in society. This type of freedom is linked with people's ability to give meaning and purpose to their own lives. The Canadian philosopher Charles Taylor pointed out that in Berlin's thought, the term 'liberty' is insufficiently problematised. Someone can be free from external constraints and still have no control over their life due to internal obstacles, such as fear or anger. Consequently, Taylor speaks of negative liberty in terms of an opportunity-concept, 'where being free is a matter of what we can do, of what it is open to us to do, whether or not we do anything to exercise this option'.[4] Positive liberty, on the other hand, is an exercise-concept: the greater people's ability is to take responsible life decisions, the more freedom they experience. This means that the central problem of freedom as an exercise-concept is whether a person is in a position to effectively carry out their plans.

As making citizens actively responsible for their own lives is not an unconditional process, I will elaborate on the term 'liberty' a little more. One the one hand, the participatory society is full of slogans like 'grass-roots', 'on your own feet', 'taking charge', 'independence', 'people power' and 'giving citizens a say' – a whole lot of upbeat terms designed to convey that playing a more active role performing public duties and running services for the common good gives citizens more control over their lives. A well-known example of this are WhatsApp groups through which the police can be notified of any suspicious activities in a given area. At the same time, however, as I have shown in the previous chapters, the government has become more suspicious of citizens, regarding them as an intrinsic risk factor that needs to be kept in check with ever more surveillance and control in the form of CCTV cameras, stop and search operations and area bans. This has made government policy extremely ambiguous: while preaching the virtues of citizens taking responsibility, it is monitoring their every move. Put bluntly, the message that the government conveys is 'we promise positive security, but provide mainly negative security'.

But what is most vital at this point in time is that the transition from welfare state to participatory society be accompanied by serious debate. Some believe that one reason for the introduction and growth of civic participation is that the welfare state has become unviable in financial and economic terms, and that the government is looking for ways of cutting costs. In that scenario, the government uses civic participation as a tool to control citizens and make them work for free, for instance by involving residents in improving liveability in their neighbourhood. Others view it as a chance to reduce the democratic deficit between citizens' expectations of democracy on the one hand and their actual experiences of it on the other. In short, a participatory society can equally be interpreted cynically, as a neoliberal economic measure, and in a more positive light, as a way of finding out how to give citizens responsibility for their own living environment on a local level.

Filthy litter

I was a member of Neighbourhood Takes Charge North Rieder for two years, to find out what issues the residents of Hillesluis were most concerned about. At the very first meeting, the council liaison officer asked us to compile a list of the three most pressing problems the neighbourhood faced, and what we wanted the police and council to focus on most. The residents present agreed unanimously that the neighbourhood's most urgent problems were (1) rubbish left beside the communal bins, (2) speeding cars and (3) a lack of parking spaces. Despite being exposed to drug dealing and violence on a daily basis, the members of NTC prioritised tackling public nuisance offences and deterioration of the neighbourhood over reducing serious crime – 'backyard problems', as one local resident called these top three issues. Broken televisions, burst bin liners, empty beer cans, food waste, littered leaflets and rubbish dumped beside the containers were the greatest source of irritation. Not only did the litter attract vermin, the residents felt it had become symbolic of a greater problem: the deterioration of the neighbourhood's image. Jocelyn, who had lived in the neighbourhood for a decade, told me with some irritation, 'When a neighbourhood is kept clean, people enjoy living there more. But there's a spot just around the corner from here where it's always filthy – driving past, you'd think you're in a slum.'

Not that the council was complacent about the litter – on the contrary, the residents in NTC agreed that it did everything to keep the neighbourhood clean. So why was it so dirty? Cynically, the answer was, 'The real problem is the attitude of the people living in Hillesluis.' The Dutch members of the committee pointed the finger at the community's foreign residents, who 'eat a lot', and they were irritated by other residents' casual attitude to littering. 'They'll toss anything on the street with the excuse that "it'll be cleaned up anyway".' The Hillesluis participation agent confirmed there was an attitude problem in the neighbourhood. 'People here like to pass the buck – they'll say, "I don't have to do that myself, that's the government's job".'

The thinking behind NTC is to give citizens the chance to prompt the council and police to tackle problems in the neighbourhood, and to explore what they themselves can do to solve the problems. On several occasions during my visits, the council liaison officer asked the residents to come up with suggestions to solve the issues raised. I noticed the term 'participatory society' was often used during the meetings, as when the council official explained to the residents that 'We are entering a participatory society. This means all of us need to become more hands-on.' The practical implications of this became clear during the ensuing discussion as to how and by whom the rubbish problem should be tackled, when the council official called on the residents to monitor the litter in their neighbourhood themselves. They rose to the challenge. At the next meeting, Jocelyn announced that he had kept track of how often rubbish was dumped next to the communal bins on Slaghek Street, while Sven had taken pictures of the rubbish. They found out that not just local residents were leaving their rubbish beside the bins, but that shops regularly did the same thing. City management responded by promising to keep an eye on the bins between 5 and 10 p.m., but that did not improve the situation.

Next, the members of NTC decided to confront littering residents in the street, but the results were again disappointing. One resident said the people she talked to sent her away with a flea in her ear: 'You're a newcomer, I've lived here for 20 years.' Another member shared a similar experience trying to tell people to pick up after their dogs and being told off for 'Betraying your own people.' The members also launched an initiative setting up two waste disposal containers between 1 and 4.30 p.m., for residents to put their rubbish in. Among the potential issues raised in the course of setting up the initiative, which took almost a year, the biggest problem was that many of the residents did not speak Dutch very well and did not know what was going on in the neighbourhood. The committee decided to distribute leaflets and put up posters to announce the container initiative, 'Ideally in seven languages', as Mieke commented pointedly. Ultimately, however, the containers also failed to get rid of the litter, as more waste was taken out of them than put inside.

To solve the problem once and for all, the residents finally proposed to replace the communal bins on the central reservation on Slaghek Street with underground containers; a proposal that soon proved difficult to implement. For one thing, the council would not permit underground containers on the grounds that the central reservation officially functioned as a green belt. Nor was it alone in opposing the residents' initiative, the landscape architects who had designed the green belt were also set against the underground containers, but it was the council's official reaction that angered and bemused the residents the most, as they did not think the central reservation was very green at all. 'Even dogs give it a wide berth', Richard seethed.

Street Takes Charge

Who sits around the table at NTC and who is missing? Are those on the committee truly representative of their neighbourhood, which consists to a significantly higher part of non-Western immigrants than the rest of Rotterdam? In other words, how do you facilitate super-diversity? Both the residents and the council acknowledged the difficulty of putting together a committee that is truly representative of Hillesluis, and most of the members of NTC are white Dutch people. 'I would love to see mothers of Turkish or Moroccan families in NTC', Lise argued, 'they know everything that goes on in the neighbourhood.' Several people told me that many residents were reluctant to get involved in council initiatives in the neighbourhood. 'The make-up of this NTC committee is very Dutch', commented Ed, who had lived in Hillesluis for over half a century. 'It's very hard to motivate the other residents to join. They don't want to get involved in anything. It's the same when you organise an event. They keep to their own groups, their own festivities, all their own things.' Local police officer Teck responded that he had made efforts to get other sections of the population involved in NTC, including the Turkish community. 'No luck though. They're just not interested,' he said, with visible disappointment.

According to Melek, a participation agent of the DOCK foundation, the fact that chiefly Dutch residents were involved in NTC was by no means unique to Hillesluis. During our conversation in the local community centre, she told me that the neighbourhoods with the largest immigrant populations also had the most Dutch members in NTC. She believed this was because Dutch people had a greater need for a platform to voice their grievances than immigrants. When immigrants complained, they usually did so among themselves. According to the council officials, the Dutch-Turkish community had a cast-iron internal network, and not much interest in the outside world. As a result, residents did not tend to stray far outside their own groups, creating inward-looking ethnic clusters in the neighbourhood. The question is, however, whether a truly proportional representation of the neighbourhood should always be the aim. For while the residents sitting on NTC may not have been an exact representation of their neighbourhood, our street survey showed that the problem they flagged up as a top priority – rubbish and littering – did reflect the neighbourhood's view. In other words, a limited descriptive representativeness need not always be at the expense of substantive representativeness.

The aim was to make NTC a household name in Hillesluis, though the survey revealed that the initiative was in fact almost or completely unknown. Barely 9% of residents surveyed said they had heard of the initiative, and only five of those were familiar with its three top priority problems. The percentage of people surveyed in the street who said they knew about NTC, though at almost 20% somewhat higher than in the questionnaire, was still very low. The reason why NTC was so unknown among residents is thought to be primarily a problem of communication. 'All the leaflets about NTC are written in Dutch', Sven pointed out, 'but this is a largely Turkish neighbourhood. Write the leaflets in Turkish and you'll reach the first generation, too. They are retired, with plenty of time on their hands, and they can motivate the younger generation'.

There was another, subtler problem. Several residents wondered if the NTC format was even suitable for the Hillesluis neighbourhood. Melek mentioned it during our conversation. She did not believe that people there were keen on projects in which they were expected to take such an active part, listing problems and tackling them themselves. 'All they want', she said, 'is to file a complaint with the authorities and hope they take action. They don't want to take on responsibility. They want a complaints committee, not a participatory committee.' Put differently, the residents did not in fact have any interest in being given administrative power. What they wanted from the meetings was to vent their anger and frustration at the government. Many residents asked for nothing more. They were glad that NTC provided a platform for them to be heard, but taking action themselves was a step too far.

The same problem came up in a different guise when I asked members in one-on-one interviews if they found working together with other residents a challenge, as there were various separate street projects running independently of each other in the neighbourhood. The best-know example is the Groene Blok (Green Bloc), a project in which the – mostly young – residents of Beukelaar Street joined forces to buy and fix up run-down houses in their street. It struck me as remarkable that the Green Bloc residents were not interested in taking part in NTC, and when I asked Sven about it, he explained, 'There is NTC, there are residents' organisations and there is the Green Bloc – and there is no communication whatsoever between them'. Melek agreed that the neighbourhood had a great many separate groups: 'The residents will join forces and get things done, but not on a neighbourhood level – they stay on their own block. They don't have the scope to cover the neighbourhood, only their street. Street Takes Charge ...'

Smiley: happy or angry?

Littering may have topped the list of irritants, but the subject most often discussed at NTC meetings was 'speeding'. This, I found out in my two years on the committee, was a real headache. The residents of North Rieder all had their own ideas on how to bring down the average driving speed in the neighbourhood, ranging from raising speed bumps to using laser gun speed traps. Ultimately, they settled on putting up a smiley, an electronic road sign showing a smiley face, as a definitive measure to discourage speeding. Depending on the speed of a passing car, the face wears a happy or sad expression, which the residents hoped would motivate drivers to stick to the speed limits. This way of subtly influencing subconscious behaviour is called nudging; people are gently nudged in the right direction without limiting their freedom to make a different choice.

All the residents attending the meeting agreed that the smiley could help put an end to the neighbourhood's speeding problem. To make the most effective use of the tool, the smiley was to be put up in the streets were people drove the fastest, starting on one side of the road and then switching to the other. But when this seemingly excellent idea was presented to the council, it responded with an endless list of reasons for denying the residents' request. The first one was that citizens were not authorised to put up smileys themselves, not even in a front garden or on the wall of a house. The council also argued that at about €1000 a month, the smiles were too expensive to run – especially given that city management already operated two of them in the neighbourhood. And finally, the residents were told that they had filed their request for the smiley with the wrong authority. Most of the arguments later turned out to be spurious.

City council and residents were locked in a stalemate for over a year. In their anger and frustration, the residents decided to write a letter about the matter to Mayor Aboutaleb. A month later, the smiley was again discussed at NTC, this time in the presence of the chairman of the Feijenoord district committee and the Feijenoord district manager. The residents talked about how completely bewildered they were by the whole situation. Just like any other NTC committee in Rotterdam, they had been given a budget to spend on purchasing materials or developing initiatives, and now they were told they could not use it to buy a smiley because the council would not give permission to do so. The district manager, worn down by talking in circles, promised with a sigh that he would 'look into it'. At the next meeting, the topsy-turvy bureaucratic process continued with an e-mail from city management to NTC. It attempted to explain the smiley situation but only went to heighten the residents' frustration. The e-mail read, 'First of all, we don't find it necessary that you, as a NTC committee, purchase another smiley when there are already two available in the area.' This drew comments from several residents, who believed the e-mail betrayed the city management's highly negative attitude. 'So they don't think we need a smiley', Mieke commented angrily. But further down the e-mail, city management invited the residents to 'compile a list of the roads where you would like to put the smiley'. Because of the e-mail's ambiguous message – smiley or no smiley? – the municipal officer suggested to invite the city management office to the next NTC meeting.

No sooner said than done. The next NTC meeting was attended by a representative of the council, who had no other choice than to agree to give the residents the loan of a smiley from September. She may have been speaking out of turn when she added that there was an unused smiley in storage, but it instantly discredited the claims about the tool's huge expense, and the council was at long last forced to put up a smiley in North Rieder. Had this smiley been present at the NTC meetings to reflect the emotional state of the Hillesluis residents, it would probably have been wearing a hysterical expression throughout in face of such administrative unwillingness and the miles of red tape they had to struggle through. 'I don't generally believe in conspiracy theories, but I got the distinct impression it was never the council's intention to give us a smiley, whether or not there was one sitting on the shelf', said Renée, head of De Piramide primary school and one of NTC's first members.

The whole episode left deep marks on the residents, their frustrating struggle for the smiley fuelling an underlying conviction that NTC was not given any real control in the neighbourhood. Talking about the little power they were given to get things done at NTC, Mieke's voice became agitated and emotional. 'I don't feel in charge at all. If I said, "This neighbourhood is too dreary, let's put up flower boxes everywhere," it wouldn't happen. I don't have that power. The council will simply say, it's not allowed, it can't be done.' Other members, equally unable to put their accumulated anger and frustration into perspective, told me their trust in the council had been undermined. Ed told me:

> It's like banging your head against a brick wall. It really is. That's why so many people give up. We decided we'd buy our own smiley because we knew it would take a year and a half or so before we'd get one from the council, and that they'd only take it down again after three months. Next thing we know, city management comes to our NTC meeting and within a month, that thing is up and running. Ridiculous, but that's the way it works. The authorities do whatever they like.

Sven even quit NTC because of the smiley; he preferred leaving the committee to keeping on bottling up his anger and frustration. 'Why leave over this?', I asked him, in his small living room. He reflected silently for a few moments, then said in a voice trembling with fury:

> We write a letter to the council and all of a sudden, it turns out city management has had one of these things going spare for years. It was just one huge last straw for me. If the council had an extra smiley lying around, why didn't they say so at once?

The Rotterdam yokel quarter

On a deeper level, the committee members' anger and frustration was also caused by an overly optimistic notion of the Hillesluis residents' ability to take charge. Countless policy documents on active citizenship assume that all citizens are able to competently act on behalf of the public good, based on the premise set out by advocates of the participatory society that citizens are all highly educated and able to analyse and solve problems, and to rationally present these problems to the authorities. Remarkably, the term 'citizen' is never problematised. The 'citizen' is invariably portrayed as a right-minded person happy to devote their time to the issue of improving liveability. However, basing a participatory society on such hypothetical model citizens also raises serious questions. The residents actually taking part in NTC were not that eloquent, as one member illustrated by describing the discussions as 'all spit and no polish'. Other members agreed they found it hard to tackle problems themselves or in consultation with the council and police. Lise said:

> I think that NTC's main task should be to organise social events like treasure hunts through the neighbourhood or a guided tour on the history of the area. That's what we're good at. Not the other things. Take the drugs problem, for example. What can we do about that? We can raise it with the council, but that's about all. The same goes for speeding. Surely this is a matter for the police.

When it takes the residents a year to get a speeding smiley, which they are then only allowed to use under the conditions imposed by the council, it makes you wonder just how much red tape the members of NTC have to get through. It also raises the question whether the initiative, meant to strengthen the brittle relationship between citizens and government rather than undermining it, is not in itself a fertile breeding ground for hysteria. The residents' main expectation is engagement with the council. Next on the list is having a say, followed in third place by receiving financial means to buy such tools as the smiley. It is hardly surprising then that they felt their complaints were not being heard and that the council was endlessly testing their patience. During the meetings, I watched residents deal with this in different ways; some quietly channelled their anger and frustration and became passive, while others got more and more fired up and angry about the council's obstinacy, fuelling the increasingly hysterical mood of the monthly meetings.

I will discuss later how feelings of loss of control and self-respect can pave the way to hysteria. First, I would like to take a look at the citizens' administrative and operational power of perseverance, and ask whether it is always sufficient for scaling the government's bureaucratic bastions. The residents sitting on the NTC committee told me they did not feel they had the power to implement the changes they would have liked to see – mainly because they did not know how, as 'the city hall is in the city centre, not here', and because 'we lack the knowledge and experience to get things done ourselves'. In other words, the residents' expertise was based on their experiences with the neighbourhood's problems, not on policies to actually tackle these problems. I noticed the same thing at one of the NTC meetings. When the community liaison officer called for a volunteer to lead the way in raising awareness of NTC, one of the residents answered frankly, 'We're an anarchistic bunch. Don't go expecting too much from us.'

Low-skilled residents generally struggle to take responsibility for social problems in the way they should according to the principles of a participatory society. By comparison, such wealthy Rotterdam neighbourhoods as Hillegersberg and East Kralingen, where the higher-income segment of the population lives, have plenty of civilian clout. Their well-off, highly educated, hip white residents know all the right people and are usually perfectly capable, through education or experience, of standing their ground against civil servants and other authorities, as I gathered from interviewing Hillesluis residents. 'South Rotterdam is the city's yokel quarter', Ed told me. 'People in Hillegersberg think nothing of writing letters, calling the police or confronting someone on the street. Hardly anyone here does that'. Jocelyn argued:

> Whether or not your voice is heard depends to a large part on where you live. Take the example of the underground containers – it took almost three years to have them put up because the landscape architects didn't want anyone spoiling the design of their green area.

The residents came up with various explanations for the passive stance in their neighbourhood, little education and little time being the most frequently named. Another key factor was a lack of what Robert Putnam calls bridging social capital, that is, making connections with people who have very different skill sets and knowledge.[5] 'Many residents work night shifts on the docks or in construction', Lise explained. 'They don't have friends in accounting firms who can write letters for them.'

It is remarkable that a policy aimed at encouraging people to participate in improving liveability does not differentiate between the various neighbourhoods and their residents. Any city of a certain size is not a single society but a wide variety of different ones living side by side, and there are even marked differences among residents of the same neighbourhood. Most of the Hillesluis residents face other, bigger problems such as unemployment, debt and domestic violence. This makes it hard for the residents of socially deprived neighbourhoods such as these to participate fully, for as the district council worker told me:

> People in this neighbourhood spend all day just trying to survive. They're not going to jump at the chance to make a meaningful contribution to their living environment. People have enough on their plates and can't really take on much more; they can't cope, it's too difficult.

Melek, a participation agent of the DOCK foundation, explained the problem:

> I think that a panel like NTC only works in places where residents are already quite articulate, have plenty of skills and are not afraid of taking responsibility. They know how to stand their ground and get their way. People in neighbourhoods like Hillesluis have neither the skills nor the extensive network to get anything done. They even lack such basic skills as writing an e-mail or sticking to an agreement.

These findings are not new. They are recurring lessons the government has yet to learn. Essentially, they mean that in order to take citizens seriously, the government needs to recognise that not everyone has equal abilities to participate in society. Not every citizen finds it easy to confront a group or is able to write a letter to the mayor of Rotterdam. The one-size-fits-all approach of NTC ignores fundamental differences between individuals and neighbourhoods, which casts doubt on the project's real contribution to rebuilding citizens' confidence in the government. As all of this goes to show, freedom of choice is not the same as the ability to choose.

Participation minus information equals frustration

On my visit to Lise, one of the neighbourhood's most engaged residents, I put the question to her why NTC achieved so few tangible results. Sitting at her kitchen table, she reflected in silence for a long time, carefully choosing her words. 'At every meeting, we talk about problems we all agree are real', she said after a while, 'but we never come to any solutions'. It galled her that everyone thought in terms of problems instead of solutions. 'Everything's bad, nothing's ever good. I try to look on the bright side, but don't always succeed.' She felt that all too often, NTC took her in a direction she did not want to go. Not that there was not plenty of room for improvement in Hillesluis. There was poverty, decay, illiteracy, early school leaving, unemployment and insecurity. All these things made Hillesluis into what it was, but, she believed, 'A positive attitude would work wonders.' The members of NTC may have failed in that respect, but to Lise, the council and police were really to blame.

The NTC members I talked to regularly told me they felt that the residents lacked the knowledge and experience to get things done. 'We get stuck on issues like rubbish, dog shit and badly parked cars, and never really get any further than everyone venting their own little grievances. It's a vicious circle. It's always the same, we get nothing done', Mieke, a resident since 1983, said. In a long conversation with Renée, I asked her about the cause of this. The question seemed to throw her off guard for a minute, but then she said, 'I can't read people's minds. Of course they want to solve their problems and improve their neighbourhood, but they don't know how and aren't getting much help in the process.' She added, more softly, 'Whether the council is consciously letting this happen – we do live in a participatory society these days – I can't tell. But nothing gets done. This NTC committee needs far more guidance.'

All residents agreed that it would be enormously helpful if the council and police provided more information on the major problems the neighbourhood faced, and gave them some indication of the solutions needed to deal with these problems successfully. 'We have no idea of what is possible', Mieke said, looking back at the past couple of years of NTC:

We don't have enough information to take control. In Spangen, they've tackled the drugs problem, in Vreewijk, empty properties. What was their approach? What exactly have they done? How did they do it? Are there other neighbourhoods that have dealt with loitering adolescents, for example? It would at least give you an idea of the possibilities.

The residents had plenty of practical ideas to improve the council's role. 'I think we need a lot more guidance from the council', one resident said, and everyone agreed that police officer Teck, especially, should play a far more active part in NTC. 'All he does now is listen', Lise said. 'It would be much better if he could tell us about the situations he's encountered in the past month, and how they've been resolved.' The same held true for other council workers. 'Their entire job revolves around this neighbourhood. They notice different things than we do because they look at the neighbourhood from a different perspective. What I would like, is more information on what is actually going on.' The residents may have wanted more information so they could take charge, but the local policeman had a different view. 'I deliberately keep information from them because I don't want to worry them unnecessarily', he explained during our conversation in the local community centre:

> NTC is meant to make the neighbourhood 'clean, intact and safe', not to make its residents anxious. It wouldn't be very helpful if I told them how many people we've arrested and how many burglaries have been committed. What does help, is to find out whether some of the complaints that residents have are justified, such as cars driving too fast on certain roads.

The municipal officer shared Teck's view that citizens should not be burdened with the big problems in the neighbourhood, which would only fuel panic and fear and lead to more emotional, even hysterical scenes, including shouting and screaming during the meetings. 'In my experience, the group is not ready to be given very much information about the neighbourhood's problems', he argued:

> As far as I can tell, only two of the members are capable of taking part in the discussion. All the others stay on the sideline, hoping they won't be asked any difficult questions. I'm afraid that if I showed up with a list of problems to discuss in more depth, a kind of top 10, it would only drive members away. People in areas like this don't have a high level of education.

The authorities' decision not to inform the members of NTC of problems in the neighbourhood is symbolic of the classic relationship between government and people, in which citizens are considered a nuisance. Power operates top-down in this system, which is argued to run counter to citizens' interests. This is regrettable, because for citizens to actually participate, it is vital they be well-informed. If not, they are left feeling they have no input in the way problems are approached in their neighbourhood. And participation without information leads only to frustration and anger. Or as Renée put it:

> If you ask me, NTC isn't about the neighbourhood taking charge at all. Is "taking charge" even the right term? Wouldn't 'Neighbourhood Puts in its Pennyworth' be better? If we are really meant to be in charge, well, that hasn't been my experience. More like 'Neighbourhood on the Sideline'.

The consequence of this all was that the growing anger and frustration of many members eventually made them drop out of the committee. In its heyday, NTC North Rieder counted a dozen members. At one point, only three turned up at the meeting, where they were faced with an impressive platoon made up of council workers, police, city management and social organisations.

Conclusion

At first glance, the Hillesluis residents' frustration and anger about the smiley and littering issues may seem trivial, and hardly indicative of a huge chasm between citizens and government. Nor can it be said that the council dismissed the problems in Hillesluis out of hand. The obstacles and red tape the residents had to overcome to find a solution to the neighbourhood's littering and speeding problems are certainly annoying, but no more than that. Yet all of this conceals a larger issue. The government's NTC program sends out contradictory messages that are confusing to the residents. Talking about trust is not the same as actually trusting. By which I mean that government policy undermines its own credibility if residents are told to take more responsibility, only for any actual initiatives developed by the same residents to be thwarted. The smiley symbolises this. When citizens see initiatives like that not being implemented, they find it hard to trust the government in return. The government wants that trust, but it will have to take the residents' input seriously in order to get it. Otherwise, disagreements between citizens and government are perceived as problematic or even insurmountable. In *Das Tabu der Virginität* (The Taboo of Virginity) from 1917, Freud called this 'the narcissism of small differences': relatively minor problems are given exaggerated importance and are eventually blown up into fundamental, unresolvable issues.

Sociologically speaking, while hysteria is typically discussed in emotional terms – as an obstacle to be overcome – it nevertheless has very real consequences in everyday life. As I have shown, the NTC members' hysteria was caused by feelings of powerlessness to respond to the council's expectations in a manageable, controlled manner. When members feel they cannot meet the requirements set out for them, they snap. This is usually the tipping point at which interacting emotions like frustration and anger can suddenly merge together, which resulted in hysterical scenes at the NTC meetings with the local government, including shouting and screaming. This chapter has shown that policy-makers' intuitive tendency to dismiss hysteria as a completely irrational phenomenon that no right-minded citizen should engage in is not just incorrect but also unwarranted, since the emotions that have caused the hysteria are genuine. In Chapter 8, I will examine hysteria's standard ingredients, which many people are prone to.

But there are other factors at play. Taking a closer look at the participatory society, we find that it exhibits countless anarchistic traits – without, however, bearing that name. I am not referring to anarchism as a political system, but as a form of human interaction, and as something that has been taking place for a long time between people who know and care for each other. For one thing, the advent of the participatory society brought the view to public attention that the neighbourhoods should be looked to for solutions to local problems rather than the government. The example of residents taking action to tackle problems in their own neighbourhood fits seamlessly into a long anarchistic tradition that aims at organising a society outside of the nation state and the market economy. But the government has shown a marked difficulty in dealing with citizens who want more say in their own lives and demand more independence. In other words, citizens are free to be as independent as they like, as long as they do what the government wants.

Calling all of this depressing would be an understatement – it is indicative of our entrenched belief that society will turn into a battlefield the moment government takes a back seat. The American TV series *The Walking Dead*, set in a world after a zombie apocalypse, illustrates this perfectly. At a moment when the world has been turned on its head, providing a unique chance to start with a blank slate, the fate of humanity is again turned over to the conventional authorities when the policemen Rick Grimes and Shane Walsh are put at the head of a group of survivors who set out to build up a new society far away from the bloodthirsty zombies. How did Vladimir Lenin put it again? 'Trust is good, control is better.'

Notes

1   The research performed here was carried out by means of in-depth interviews, observations at the monthly NTC meetings, perceptions in the Rotterdam Hillesluis neighbourhood, document research, and a survey. In total, 12 in-depth interviews were held with the members of the NTC committee, including the residents, local police officer, urban management official, participation agent of the DOCK foundation, and the founder of NTC, Hans Hoekman. The interviews varied in length from one hour to almost two hours. In the interviews, I asked the residents about their opinion on the effectiveness of NTC and whether it had increased their trust in the police and council. I also wanted to know if the security issues discussed by NTC had been addressed and whether they had noticed any improvements. Finally, I asked the residents to what degree they believe they were capable of actually exercising their freedom of choice. The survey was filled in by 58 men and 63 women. In proportion with the make-up of the neighbourhood, Dutch ($n = 40$) and Dutch-Turkish residents

(n = 38) were the most represented. The age of the citizens who took the survey ranged from 14 to 87 years. In a questionnaire consisting of rating scale questions, they were asked among other things about their familiarity with the NTC programme, and whether they had noticed improvements in their neighbourhood with regard to the problems outlined by the committee.

2 Skogan (2006).
3 Berlin (1969).
4 Taylor (1979, p. 177).
5 Putnam (2000).

Chapter 7

Race riots in Rotterdam

Introduction

No other subject touches the nerve of hysteria quite as much as that of immigration into one's country. Stories about asylum seekers and refugees have dominated the headlines for years, claiming that all refugees are 'rapists' and 'terrorists' and pose the biggest threat to Western countries since the Second World War. This exacerbates the already heightened tensions in society between supporters and opponents of refugee centres. People are particularly opposed to asylum seekers being housed close to their own homes – in municipalities where asylum centres are opened, mayors and other council officials receive death threats, and dozens of people have been arrested for storming emergency refugee shelters. When it comes to the influx of refugees, Twitter and Facebook seem to be divided into two camps: the 'enraged citizens' and the 'do-gooders'. Comments on these social media platforms can get so grim that posters are regularly charged with hate-mongering and incitement to violence. The tenor of the discussion about receiving refugees is remarkably hysterical, the general noise being riddled with toxic tweets, from highly articulate representatives of a supercharged outrage. 'Let's all go down the town hall, get those bastards to sod off', as one angry citizen wrote in a tweet that got over one hundred likes.

Nor is the political debate on the subject exactly marked by a confident, composed tone. The populist parties of numerous countries are upholding their election promise to bar immigrants from entering the country. Besides Donald Trump, the Italian, Polish and Hungarian leaders have also closed their countries' borders. In the Dutch Second Chamber, basic instincts consistently triumph over facts and nuances. According to political commentator Charlie Sykes, democracy has become a 'binary tribal world, where everything is at stake, everything is in play',[1] and where emotions run so high, debate becomes focused on controversial statements rather than on substantive issues and solutions. Anything to get attention. 'Want fewer asylum seekers? Leave it to us', right-wing parties promise. But they have not been alone in recent years in saying that the borders should be closed – other parties also want to call a halt to immigration and deport illegal immigrants with immediate effect, and bolster these demands by continuously bombarding voters with apocalyptic visions of the demise of our society at the hands of hordes of illiterate, non-integrable 'fortune seekers' flooding the country.

The hysterical tenor of the political debate is all the more remarkable given that governments and politicians are supposed to act rationally and not allow themselves to be swept away by an excess of emotions. Rational political behaviour has been considered a vital feature of a perfectly functioning democracy since the Enlightenment, with reason and the unambiguous language of figures and statistics as its key elements. In fact, politicians could choose to view the influx of newcomers in a different light, for instance as a solution for labour shortages – the IT sector, among others, has been struggling with staff shortages for years despite various recruitment initiatives. But such a perspective reflects a short-term view that does little justice to the far longer history of hysteria in the Western world, and which disregards the complexity of such social problems as the arrival of immigrants in the Netherlands.

Given that hysteria has a detrimental effect on long-term memory, it might be a good idea to go back in time to the violent disturbances of August 1972 that would become known as the race riots of the Rotterdam Afrikaander neighbourhood. It was the first time the Netherlands experienced what would colloquially become known as 'Turk riots'. On a sunny Wednesday in South Rotterdam, a knife fight between residents helping a Dutch woman move house and members of a Turkish community living in the same building led to disturbances that would last almost a week. This incident and the discussions it ignited shed an interesting light on the issue of immigration hysteria. Why did the riots erupt in the Afrikaander neighbourhood? What caused the public mood to swing so suddenly? How did politicians react to the turbulent events of August 1972? In other words, what can we learn from history that will help us better to understand the current hysteria over the arrival of immigrants?

Angry mob in the Afrikaander neighbourhood

On 9 August 1972, the first race riot in the Netherlands broke out in South Rotterdam, between Dutch and Turkish residents.[2] The conflict was sparked when an argument between the 26-year-old Dutch single mother Gerda and her Turkish landlord Mehmet got out of hand in the Afrikaander neighbourhood. The woman, who was in arrears, asked the police whether she was allowed to prevent Mehmet from seizing her belongings. Mehmet had told her a couple of days earlier that he would cancel her debt if she went to bed with him. When the police made it clear that the landlord would not be able to recover the owed rent unless he started civil proceedings, the woman decided to move house.

At 5.11 p.m. on the day of the move, Gerda and Mehmet got into a huge argument at 10A Goede Hoop Street, and by the time the police arrived at 6.23 p.m., a large crowd had gathered in front of the house. Inside, three neighbours who were helping the woman to move had started a fight with four Turkish inhabitants of the house. The police found that three injured Dutch men had been stabbed by the Turks during the fight, and learned, among other things, that the landlord had pulled out a knife after furniture belonging to him had been thrown out of the window and set on fire. While the police arrested the four Turkish men on the fourth floor, a crowd of people gathered on the street to see what was going on. The police had to form a cordon to take the Turkish suspects to the police car.

They were soon surrounded by almost 500 angry residents chanting racist slogans and shouting that they would lynch the immigrant workers. At this point, according to the report of the Rotterdam police, the officers fired a warning shot to keep the 'overwrought and aggressive' crowd at a distance, which allowed them to reach the police car with the suspects. But peace was not restored to the neighbourhood with the departure of the police; on the contrary, the same evening, more windows were smashed in houses where immigrant workers live, as well as those of the Turkish Ankara Café on Paarl Street, and the Turkish landlord's car was tipped over. The next day, the disturbances in Paarl Street and Goede Hoop Street continued, with the first agitated anti-Turkish protesters gathering at around 10 a.m. At 2 p.m., the police were alerted by the district committee and told that the residents would 'probably start forming vigilante groups to be ready to crush any actions the Turks might be planning'. At this, the police decided to put ten more officers on surveillance duty, increasing the number to 30. But even this increased force could not prevent an angry mob from occupying the boarding house above the Ankara Café and throwing all the furniture out of the window from the fourth floor, including mattresses, lamps, clothes, pots and pans. The occupiers demanded that this living space be made available to Dutch people again, threatening to take further action if it was not. Meanwhile, things went from bad to worse. Fire-bombs and stones were thrown through the windows of various boarding houses, signs were put up saying 'for rent for Dutch people only', and Paarl Street was renamed Hollandse Street (Dutch Street). Police presence was increased further, to 42 officers.

On Friday 11 August, Labour alderman for public housing Henk Jettinghoff and the chief of police visited the occupied boarding house, assuring the occupiers that they would not be arrested by the police. In response, the protest committee nailed a pamphlet to the boarded-shut window of an evacuated Turkish cafe, calling on people not to take any further action after the occupations on Wednesday and Thursday. The pamphlet read, 'Be reasonable, go home, because everything that is wrecked from now on will only harm our cause.' The committee also appealed to the residents to stop using violence. None of this had much effect, however, as crowds of rioters poured into the neighbourhood and the disturbances continued in the street, where a new mob had gathered and was chanting loud and clear anti-Turkish slogans. More windows of Turkish boarding houses were smashed, now in the adjacent South Rotterdam neighbourhoods Bloemhof and Hillesluis. The atmosphere was especially grim on Wagen Street and Slaghek Street in Hillesluis. Armed with truncheons, the police charged the crowd in an effort to disperse it, while people pried cobblestones and bricks out of the streets and hurled them at patrol cars. The police reported that the scene on the street had turned 'from the unrest of anti-Turkish protests into a common riot, with most of the rioters being young people between 15 and 25 years of age'. 'You'd think it was New Year's Eve', a police spokesman commented.

On the weekend, hooligans and riot tourists arrived from other parts of Rotterdam and other cities to do battle with the police in the Afrikaander neighbourhood, pelting police officers with stones and wrecking patrol cars. Riot police were deployed to quell the riots for good and restore calm to the neighbourhood, but on Sunday 13 August, there were plenty more scuffles between Turkish and Dutch residents, and the police arrested 7 Turkish and 19 Dutch people for acts of public violence. With the police failing to put an end to the clashes, a group of residents decided to take it upon themselves to restore order and asked permission from the police to act as a civilian arrest squad. According to the police report, they wanted to 'take the law into their own hands and restore order to the neighbourhood with an iron fist'. Other residents wanted the police to seal off the neighbourhood in order to keep rioters out. But the police refused to honour either request, so as to disrupt everyday life as little as possible. On Monday, almost a week after the first incident, the riots were finally over.

Arrival city Rotterdam

Sociologically speaking, Rotterdam is a typical arrival city. Its economic growth after the Second World War initially attracted immigrant workers from Italy and Spain, and migrants from Turkey and Morocco started arriving in the mid-1960s to become construction and dock workers. The Turkish community saw a particularly fast growth in the 1960s – while Rotterdam's register of foreign nationals counted 19 Turkish residents in 1961, that number had reached 5051 a decade later.

The term 'arrival city' was coined by British-Canadian journalist Doug Saunders in his 2011 bestseller *Arrival City*, a study into the major migratory flows from rural to urban areas, in which he examines around 30 arrival cities around the world and reaches a number of remarkable conclusions about the comparatively poor neighbourhoods in which newcomers settle. Saunders's most important finding is that the existence of such neighbourhoods does not automatically lead to extra problems – no need to bring in the bulldozers and level them to the ground. Of course there can be no comparison between the Rotterdam South Afrikaander neighbourhood and the slums of Nairobi or Mumbai, but whatever the differences of these arrival cities, Saunders believes that the positive socio-economic processes taking place among the newcomers are the same. For all the residents are seeking a better life in work, education for their children, a shop or restaurant of their own, and they all connect with compatriots who went before them in the neighbourhoods they settle in — 'slums of hope', as Saunders calls them — creating the kind of community that enables them to take their first step up the social ladder. After a while, many of the residents are able to move to a better neighbourhood, and a new generation of newcomers take their place. As a result, the neighbourhood may stay poor but its residents will not.

After a large part of the city was destroyed in the Second World War, the 'planned city' became a dominant ideal in Rotterdam, as is evident from the numerous visions for the future presented just after the war, which emphasised the importance of forging tightly knit urban communities of people who share a real connection. The urban development and sociocultural study *De stad der toekomst, de toekomst der stad* (The City of the Future, the Future of the City) from 1946, for example, proposes that Rotterdam be built up of areas of approximately 20,000 residents with strong ties to their neighbourhood. This plan views the residential area as a link between individual living space and society as a whole. It includes maximising social cohesion by providing each neighbourhood with facilities such as allotments, sports grounds, schools, green areas and medical and social care, and is dominated by classic biopolitical strategies focused on regulating the living conditions of the people of Rotterdam. The report states, for example, that neighbourhood cohesion must fulfil an 'extremely pedagogical role so as to raise and maintain the physical, medical and hygiene standards of the population, and to make sure people are sufficiently informed and supported, socially and pedagogically'.

But despite its intention of turning all of Rotterdam into a planned city after the Second World War, the city council spent the first decades after liberation concentrating on rebuilding the bombed centre of the city, where 24,000 houses, 2400 shops and around 4000 other buildings had been destroyed. Financial means being limited, funds for the construction of new houses and the expansion of residential areas outside of the centre were drastically cut. The original plan of building homes for various different income groups in Pendrecht and Zuidwijk was shelved. The council's decision not to build higher-end properties in those neighbourhoods led to a further deterioration of the local housing market, which contributed to a one-sided population profile. The other arrival neighbourhoods in South Rotterdam did not profit much from the planned-city mania sweeping the city either. Large parts of South Rotterdam sank further into decay, and the council left the original inhabitants as well as the Turkish and Moroccan newcomers to their fate. Many houses were so poorly maintained and dilapidated they became uninhabitable. On top of that, the arrival of low-skilled migrants and the deterioration of the neighbourhood were causing a great deal of social unrest. A growing number of the original residents, young families especially, moved from the working-class neighbourhoods in South Rotterdam to one of the suburbs, or left the city altogether. The houses they vacated were soon inhabited by Turkish and Moroccan guest workers, and, to a lesser degree, students.

It was not as if Rotterdam politicians did not know about the abominable living conditions in working class neighbourhoods, the decay of the houses, the lack of facilities and the general decline of the area. The question arises, however, whether the residents felt their grievances were being heard and addressed. They had complained bitterly about bad living conditions and about the council ignoring the problems in the South Rotterdam neighbourhoods for years before the poor housing of guest workers finally made it onto the agenda of the council in 1971, one year before the race riots erupted in the Afrikaander neighbourhood. In the same year, on 13 May, the Liberal Party council member Wim Baggerman called an extraordinary city council meeting in which he voiced his concern about the accommodation, social integration and support of immigrant workers in Rotterdam. Baggerman stated that there were over 18,000 foreign workers in and around the city of Rotterdam, and that he believed there were 'clear cases of blatant mismanagement where the housing of foreign workers was concerned'. In a recent example, fires breaking out in boarding houses for foreign workers had left one person dead, three injured and eight homeless, which according to Baggerman was down to the grim housing situation and the fact that the boarding houses did not meet health, safety and hygiene standards. Baggerman spoke about a boarding house in which 70 people were 'packed together in a rat trap'. He concluded that the housing of foreigners was below par and that these people were only seen as objects to be exploited. On behalf of the Liberal Party, he demanded 'better treatment [of foreigners] and that they are not to be exploited like slaves nor treated as such – or should I say, "mistreated"'.

Media hysteria

In August 1972, Rotterdam made global headlines when the Afrikaander neighbourhood residents' anger and frustration reached breaking point and escalated in riots. Newspaper and television reporters flocked to the neighbourhood looking for explanations for the riots. Had they just come out of nowhere, or could a long history of events preceding them explain their nature and scale? In fact, the Afrikaander neighbourhood riots did not come as a complete surprise. A year earlier, on 7 January 1971, the Mayor of Rotterdam Wim Thomassen stated in a speech about the year 1970 that 'the discrepancy between such areas with no housing shortage and the disadvantaged areas is growing'. Thomassen warned the council that 'resolving this issue is going to be a long struggle'. The *Rotterdams Nieuwsblad* of 27 March 1971 reported on a survey held in the old working-class neighbourhood Crooswijk showing that four out of ten of its residents were opposed to the arrival of immigrant workers, and quoted such arguments as, 'They don't belong here', 'They bring down the neighbourhood', and 'They're dirty and make too much noise'.

In June of the same year, the local Pro Guest Workers action committee (AKPG) warned of a risk of riots breaking out in the Afrikaander neighbourhood, which they compared to a ticking time bomb. According to the *Haagse Post* of 26

June 1971, 'A race riot is brewing in Rotterdam.' The Rotterdam paper *De Havenloods* also mentioned tensions in the old Rotterdam working class neighbourhoods more than once. In September 1971, protesters at a rally in West Rotterdam demanded that the government put a stop to the influx of migrant workers. In a letter to the council, the action group warned of a 'collective anxiety psychosis' triggered by the steady stream of immigrants into the city.

Covering the riots for the current affairs programme *Televizier Magazine* of the Dutch broadcaster AVRO, television reporter Jaap van Meekren said with a troubled expression, 'Rotterdam. It's not Belfast and never will be. Nor is it Berlin during Kristallnacht in 1938, but there are parallels, and that is disgrace enough.' Various people involved in the riots were interviewed on TV. Their statements clearly show that the residents felt left in the lurch by politics, and that the process of integration between various population groups in deprived areas was a slow and difficult one. One of the rioters gave the following explanation for the violent unrest:

> We're setting an example for the government to take action. I don't mind foreigners being here at all. But make them live in separate houses, so they can stay among themselves. If they live among us, you just know there'll be trouble, you can count on it. We've seen this coming for years, and now everything has come to a head.

A spokesman for the Afrikaanderwijk neighbourhood group summed up the residents' sentiments:

> Turks discriminate against the Dutch. Because when a Turk buys a property and moves in, he'll harass the people living there and do everything he can to get them to leave. So there's plenty of folks been leading normal lives in this neighbourhood for the past 30 or 40 years who have been pestered so much by the foreigners they've had to move house.

The printed press also offered its opinion. Dutch newspapers published extensive daily reports on the ongoing riots in a hysterical, frenzied tone without providing a shred of evidence of the facts. The *Reformatorisch Dagblad*, for example, wrote about 'groups of Turks armed with pistols about to take action'. Foreign interest in the riots was equally overwhelming. The Turkish papers *Milliyet* and *Hürriyet*, who publish special editions for Turks living in Belgium, Germany and the Netherlands, reported on the riots, and a *New York Times* journalist professed to be 'shocked and startled'. The *Washington Post* concluded that the 'Dutch image of tolerance [is] shattered'. A *Guardian* headline read, 'Dutch surprised by race clashes', and *The Times* wrote on 12 August 1972:

Most Brits will be surprised to hear about the race riots in Rotterdam. The incident does not fit the general image we have of the Netherlands in this country. We think of the Dutch as a rational, moderate, peace-loving, unbiased, progressive, decent, hard-working people who are always welcoming to foreigners.

Despite the diversity of warring parties on the battlefield of the Afrikaander neighbourhood, the media sided mostly with the immigrant residents in the conflict, concentrating almost exclusively on the newcomers' situation and much less on the complaints of the original residents of the old neighbourhoods. Historian Cheska Polderman wrote that 'guest workers were invariably depicted as "pitiable" while the other residents were lumped together with racists and rioters'.[3]

Reporters covering the riots were not afraid of using highly charged terms in their sensationalist reports on the turmoil raging in the neighbourhood, or of highlighting ethnic tensions and presenting them in terms of war and the Holocaust. The *Haagse Post*, for example, used the portmanteau word 'Pogrommerdam'. The message of the media could not have been clearer: a civil war was raging in South Rotterdam. TV reporter Jaap van Meekren was just as unambiguous in his conclusion, ending his report on 14 August 1972, accompanied by images of cornered boarders, with the words:

> Tomorrow or the day after, or perhaps next week, calm will return to this place. Some people will move house. Windowpanes will be replaced, houses refurnished and an investigation committee will probably be set up. But the Turkish man who collects your household rubbish or cleans oil tankers here in the port or works next to you in the factory, now suddenly has a very different impression of what we like to call his host country. The Netherlands' global reputation has been damaged. British television stations are filming this tonight. It wouldn't hurt for certain residents of Rotterdam to take a long hard look in the mirror and ask themselves what it is they see.

Quite a speech, which boils down to the message that foreigners should not be feared, but the original Dutch inhabitants of Rotterdam should be.

Heard from telegraph lines

The way in which the media create crisis events, also known as framing, is a particular speciality of such English tabloid newspapers as *The Sun, The Daily Mirror* and *The Daily Express* that are known for their own, unique view of reality. Typical features of these papers are their catchy headlines, colourful spreads with many photographs and a highly personal angle. The headlines regularly trigger hysterical reactions, and the daily dose of scandal, gossip and sensation they spread make Dutch newspapers seem like a beacon of calm by comparison. A good example of this is the social unrest that gripped England in the 1960s as a result of fights breaking out between two British youth groups, the mods and the rockers. The media viewed the mod and rocker subcultures as 'a reaction to the strict discipline of the Victorians'.[4] The mods rode around on scooters, listened ska and soul music, wore fashionable clothes and had distinctive haircuts, while the rockers liked rock music, wore black leather jackets and rode heavy motorbikes. In 1964, the two groups got into a fight in Clacton, a small seaside resort on the southeast coast of England. During the brawls, the windows of several shops and a nightclub were smashed, a number of beach huts destroyed, and a gun was fired into the air by one of the brawlers. The total damage amounted to 500 pounds. The police, caught off guard by the riots, arrested almost 100 youths for 'unruly behaviour', 'insulting an officer on duty' and 'resisting arrest'. But though the damage was limited and no excessive violence had been used, the front pages of British newspapers were full of spectacular headlines in the days that followed. Terms like 'Day of Terror' (*Daily Telegraph*), 'Wild Ones Invade Seaside' (*Daily Mirror*) and 'Youngsters Beat up Town' (*Daily Express*) dominated the headlines.

In his 1972 book *Folk Devils and Moral Panics*, Stanley Cohen refers to the riots between the mods and the rockers to introduce the concept of 'moral panic'. According to Cohen, politicians and citizen are gripped by panic when rules are violated by individuals or groups that are considered a serious threat to society, such as drug users, football hooligans or paedophiles. While giving no actual definition of what moral panic is, Cohen makes it clear in his examples that it is caused by individuals or groups whose behaviour poses a threat to fundamental social values and interests. It is aggravated by an exaggerated media emphasis, compared with more objective sources on the one hand and different, more pressing problems on the other, of the incident's implications and importance. This often leads to an excessive negative response to the deviant behaviour and to reactions like stigmatisation and exclusion of the perpetrators that are disproportionate to what has actually happened.

The etymological origin of the word 'panic' derives from the Greek *deima panikon*: fear caused by Pan. There is, however, a large gap between the mythological substrate of this adjective on the one hand and the meaning of the word 'panic' – in the sense of a sudden, overwhelming fear – on the other. The son of Hermes and the nymph Penelope, Pan was the Greek god of shepherds and their flocks. He dwelt in the darkest and most impenetrable parts of the woods and forests and was the friend and patron of hunters, fishermen, bee-keepers and shepherds and their livestock. But besides his positive role as the patron of shepherds and flocks, Pan had another, darker side. In Greek mythology, Pan is represented as half-human, half-goat with a repulsive face, horns, a goat's beard, pointy ears, a tail, goat's legs and a hairy body. He enjoyed startling people and animals and making them panic by suddenly appearing out of nowhere or making strange, terrifying sounds. Strictly speaking, any further reaction of the victim's – such as taking flight – can no longer be called panic. On the contrary, fleeing immediately after the moment of panic is a kind of rational escape that puts an end to the panic.[5] In fact, Pan may have looked monstrous, but his threats did not amount to much in practice – it was really just a lot of noise.

Moral panic is indicative of an elite's underlying fear of the prevailing morality being eroded by a subculture. It interprets a certain incident or behaviour as an assault on its existence. In this clear-cut worldview, the prevailing morality belongs to the establishment while subcultures form an opposition force. But not every reaction of a subculture makes society panic, which raises the question where the establishment's oversensitivity comes from and where such a reaction can lead. Erich Goode and Nachman Ben-Yehuda answer this question by distinguishing between five stages of moral panic: concern, hostility, consensus, disproportionality and volatility.[6] It all begins with a heightened concern about the antisocial behaviour of certain individuals or groups and its adverse effects on society. This concern is then reflected by a certain degree of hostility towards those individuals or groups, the so-called 'folk devils', who are depicted as 'evil' and 'enemies of society'. A stereotypical representation of the incident subsequently leads to a dichotomy between good and bad, which in turn strengthens what the French sociologist Émile Durkheim called the collective conscience of society. The third step, a widespread and general consensus that there is a real and serious danger, leads to a public debate, magnifying perceptions of not only the behaviour itself but also the threat it poses. This is often accompanied by a disproportionate political reaction to the actual threat. The last stage of moral panic is volatility. Moral panic vanishes as quickly as it appeared, which does not mean that it has no lasting negative effects. The debate on the reprehensible behaviour often gives rise to new laws being implemented, and moral panic tends slowly but surely to change social norms. Examples are the hippies and their struggle for more democracy, and women in the 1960s calling for equal treatment to men.

Panic or hysteria?

Cohen explains moral panic as 'the generation of diffuse normative concerns, while the successful creation of folk devils rests on their stereotypical portrayal as atypical actors against a background that is overtypical'.[7] He considers the media as the most important platform for heightened concern, and a tool for spreading panic. The idea behind this is to show that social responses to certain events or behaviours are heavily influenced by newspapers, television and the Internet. Not only do they define certain problems by controlling which topics are covered and which are not, the media also provide a platform for so-called 'moral entrepreneurs', a term coined by Howard Becker in his book *Outsiders* to describe people who take the moral high ground in order to push certain issues onto the agenda and convince others of their point of view.[8] So when Cohen speaks of moral panic, he is not saying that the entire population has shut themselves up in their homes or are running for their lives from imminent danger. Cohen uses the word 'panic' to refer to the way in which certain events and situations are represented in newspaper articles, TV reports, political debates and even laws, and the prioritisation of certain measures.

In the introduction to the third edition of *Folk Devils and Moral Panic*, Cohen lists a variety of subjects that are particularly likely to trigger a moral panic response. A case in point is violence in schools, such as the suicide of a pupil who has been bullied by others. School shootings are also frequent triggers of panic in a society, such as the shooting at Columbine High School in 1999, in which two boys murdered 12 fellow students and a teacher. Another topical example of moral panic is the supposed effect on consumers of sex and violence in popular culture, ranging from comic books to video games and from superhero movies to rap music. A regularly recurring question is whether violence in popular culture really is the harmless entertainment it is made out to be, or if there is in fact a connection between violent behaviour in adolescents and violence in movies, music and video games. Some believe that violent song lyrics increase negative feelings and aggressive behaviour, while others argue they provide adolescents with an outlet for their aggression. After the Columbine High School shooting, shock rocker and satanist Marilyn Manson was accused of inspiring the two perpetrators Eric Harris and Dylan Klebold to commit the murders.

In the mid-1980s, paedophiles became the best-known folk devils in Western society. It is hard to imagine today how different public opinion about these 'sexual monsters' was only 50 years ago, when prominent Dutch people like the psychologist Frits Bernard and Labour senator Edward Brongersma openly discussed their love for under-age children. There was also a literary tradition surrounding paedophilia, propagated by such writers as Jan Hanlo and Rudi van Dantzig, and the Dutch government was even drafting a law to legalise child pornography. Paedophilia was called the last great taboo. *De Volkskrant* headline of 9 April 1981 read, 'Paedophilia Often a Positive Experience for Child'. After an incident in Oude Pekela in the province of Groningen in 1987, however, in which dozens of children were thought to have been abducted and abused, and the beginning of the Dutroux case in Belgium in 1996, public tolerance for paedophilia decreased sharply. Sexual intercourse between adults and minors was once again considered immoral and criminal behaviour.

In the Danish film *Jagten* (2012), directed by Thomas Vinterberg, public anger flares up in a rural village when primary school teacher Lucas is falsely accused of child abuse by one of his pupils. Lucas, played brilliantly by Mads Mikkelsen, expects the misunderstanding to be cleared up quickly, but underestimates the sinister dynamics of mass hysteria that has gripped the whole village and leads the villagers to collectively hunt him down. His faithful dog is murdered, the windows of his house broken, and he is heavy-handedly removed from the supermarket. Vinterberg uses the theme of the hunt to convey a chilling story of how a community closes ranks, as if wanting to erect a wall against a common enemy, and how Lucas is slowly driven insane.

While the term 'moral panic' is useful for describing media hypes triggered by unexpected and undesirable events, which can range from sexual abuse of children to the radicalisation of Muslim youth and from violent video games to the arrival of asylum seekers, the use of the word 'panic' remains unclear.[9] In *Folk Devils and Moral Panic*, Cohen does not differentiate between panic and hysteria, indiscriminately using different terms for overreaction such as 'hysteria' and 'delusion' as if they were synonyms of each other.[10] This risks giving the impression that the concept of 'moral panic' is self-explanatory, and ignores theoretical differences between panic and hysteria. In this case, it is even more remarkable, because according to the American sociologist Neil Smelser, whom Cohen refers to several times in his book, hysteria actually lies at the base of panic. In his 1962 book *Theory of Collective Behaviour*, Smelser writes, 'Hysterical beliefs are necessary conditions for the development of the panic.'[11]

Panic is never simply panic. Although it is difficult to differentiate, in causal or in phenomenological terms, between hysteria and panic, I think that there should be a clear division between the two. According to the etymology of the word, panic is a form of sudden, overwhelming fear, triggered by a specific, concrete cause. As an example, some people panic when they see a spider. They might think the spider was about to climb up their trouser leg, and the thought makes their body's stress system kick in and results in panic. Hysteria, on the other hand, is a form of existential anxiety – an unconscious anxiety constantly present in our daily lives, which comes to the fore when we experience the feeling of losing control and which is very hard to conquer. As a result, hysteria often masks a larger conflict that leads to powerful emotions and uncontrolled behaviour in individuals. Rather than by a concrete threat ('the spider'), hysteria is triggered by an unspecified social or cultural conflict that is too large and abstract for individuals to deal with, such as the current refugee crisis. Following this line of reasoning, hysteria focuses on distant subjects that nevertheless feel very close. Freud called this the *Unheimlich* (the uncanny): the troubling intrusion of the unfamiliar into the familiar.

Uprooted and uncanny

Freud describes the uncanny as 'that class of the terrifying which leads back to something long known to us, once very familiar'.[12] The German word *Unheimlich* is hard to translate, as it combines connotations of 'homey' and 'hidden'. *Heimlich* refers to that which is familiar and known (belonging to the home), but can also mean 'suspicious' and 'surreptitious'. The negative meanings of the antonym *Unheimlich* are therefore already present in the positive term *Heimlich* itself. Both terms share the same meaning: the feeling of security in the home or family is threatened from the inside by something disturbing.

Freud's study of the uncanny was published in the autumn of 1919. Strikingly, he gives over a hundred different meanings of the term in the first four pages of his essay, as if something uncontrollable and hysterical were going on under the surface of the text. Freud based his findings on the 1906 article 'Zur Psychologie des Unheimlichen' by Ernst Anton Jentsch, who defines the uncanny as a sense of uncertainty about something unknown. But as Freud points out, this does not mean something is uncanny because it is strange and unknown. On the contrary, it is a fear that comes up when the familiar suddenly appears strange. If we ignore all psychoanalytical references to such concepts as repression, death wish and castration in Freud's text for the moment, it becomes clear why Western countries respond with hysteria to the arrival of refugees. The home no longer offers safety and security because it is threatened by an uncanny, disturbing and transnational phenomenon. In this context, the term *Heim* covers a certain space or territory, such as a neighbourhood, village or national territory, which is reflected in arguments like, 'They don't share our values', and 'They're taking all our jobs'.

But this is not the place for an extensive discourse on the uncanny. Nor does everything that is uncanny always trigger hysteria, but one aspect of it is of importance for a better understanding of immigration hysteria. Confronted with a large-scale, abstract phenomenon like mass immigration, many people who never come into contact with refugees nevertheless feel as though their safe 'home' is being invaded by strangers. It makes them feel they have lost control of their own destiny, like losing the key to your front door. We could also apply the neologism 'extimity' (*extimité*), which is a contraction of 'extern' and 'intimate', coined by Jacques Lacan to describe the strangeness at the core of everyone's intimacy. As a result of this situation, the sense of security that originates inside the womb and is etymologically linked to the Greek *hysterikos*, is in danger of slowly but surely disappearing. You could say that globalisation and a sense of security do not go well together. In the last chapter, I will discuss the way this loss of a sense of security, which begins with the umbilical cord being cut too soon, finds an outlet in hysteria.

Meanwhile at the town hall

In his opening speech on 6 January 1972, during the first council meeting of the year in which Rotterdam would be confronted with the Afrikaander neighbourhood race riots, Mayor Thomassen said, 'We have entered the year 1972 in a climate of apprehension.' Thomassen spoke of the Vietnam War and touched on the international nature of environmental issues by speaking of the awakening of global environmental awareness. In the same year, the Club of Rome drew widespread public attention with its *The Limits of Growth* report, in which the link was made for the first time between economic growth and its impact on the environment. Thomassen also announced that the population of Rotterdam had reached 670,000. He spoke of the necessity of improving public transport in the city and referred to the United States, where cities with no future were in danger of being suffocated by the lack of public transport.

On 16 March 1972, barely six months before the riots broke out, a proposal was submitted to refurbish houses in the working class Afrikaander and Oude Westen neighbourhoods. Various councillors spoke out their support, among them the Communist Party member Mr Van Zanden, who stated that 'the government's inability to adopt effective policies has forced a large part of the population to live in socially unacceptable housing in equally unacceptable neighbourhoods'. Speaking on behalf of the Labour party, Ms Molenaar welcomed the proposal, saying that 'a large part of the living space currently available to people in this city is effectively uninhabitable'. But the alderman responsible, labour member Mr Jettinghoff, tempered the city council's expectations, saying it was a difficult task which he did 'not feel confident will be accomplished in the near future'. The reason for this was because the houses were privately owned rather than belonging to a housing association or council housing. Two months later on 25 May 1972, the abject state of housing in Rotterdam working class neighbourhoods was again discussed. This time, Labour member Mr Van Hattem spoke up on a proposed moving cost reimbursement programme for residents who voluntarily vacated their homes. He mentioned the situation in Rubroek, a neighbourhood in Crooswijk, which looked 'as if it were ravaged by war. There are empty windows, burnt-out houses and condemned buildings.' In response to questions of the council, the councillor announced that 500,000 Dutch guilders had been earmarked for moving cost reimbursements.

On 17 August 1972, the day after the race riots ended, Mayor Thomassen made the following statement during the city council afternoon session:

> The events that took place in and around the Afrikaander neighbourhood between Wednesday 9 August until last night have been a bitter disappointment to us. Those past few days were marked by disturbances, aggressive behaviour, vandalism, tension and fear.

The shocking events in the Afrikaander neighbourhood clearly left deep scars on the Rotterdam authorities. It felt as if the established order had been shaken to its foundations, as Thomassen made plain in his passionate denouncement of the riots in which he referred to the Rotterdam Enlightenment thinkers Hugo Grotius and Desiderius Erasmus:

> Erasmus gazes down into the city from above the middle window of the town hall, while the north-east corner of the building is adorned by Hugo Grotius. If they had witnessed what happened in the city that was once theirs, they – like us – would have been ashamed.

But in remarkable contrast to reports on television and newspaper headlines, Thomassen refused to lay the blame for the riots on just one party. Instead, he held Turkish and Dutch residents alike responsible for the disturbances:

Examining the facts, we must conclude that there were Turkish people who behaved badly and Dutch people who behaved badly, and that the resulting conflicts escalated into riots and disruption, which made restoring and maintaining order an imperative.

Referring to the police report drawn up after the riots, Thomassen listed a variety of possible causes. The main cause, he told the overcrowded council meeting, were 'problems connected with the arrival and accommodation of migrant workers, especially with regard to housing, the establishment of boarding houses and the accumulation of such boarding houses in certain neighbourhoods'. As it transpired, the migrant workers the city had attracted after the Second World War were by that time living in the most degrading circumstances. The concentration of overpopulated boarding houses was especially high in the city's old neighbour-hoods, where on some streets as many as one in 16 houses was a boarding house. Most of them were owned by rack renters of Turkish origin trying to squeeze in as many Moroccan, Turkish and southern European tenants as possible. The rooms, which were often unheated, were apparently shared by several tenants who took turns sleeping in a single bed.

Testosterone politics

It will have struck anyone attending the Rotterdam Council meetings at the time that the language used bore no resemblance to the hysterical tone adopted by the national media. The politicians in the town hall of Rotterdam did not use inflammatory, emotional language, and irrationality, pathos or hysterical witch hunts were not tolerated. No amplification spiral – in which various phases of moral panic overlap and intensify each other – was set in motion, no Freudian projection of fears onto a folk devil took place. The councillors spoke of the race riots in the Afrikaander neighbourhood in measured and nuanced language, framing their account of the riots in terms of reconciliation and union rather than war, battle and hostility. One indication of this is that the representatives of the political parties refused to speak of a racial conflict, instead interpreting the riots in a socio-economic framework. The Labour Party, for example, took the view that 'the tensions and difficulties did not originate in racial discrimination – this eruption was caused by inadequate policies'. Labour member Van der Have spoke of a conflict in which 'worker turns against worker'. He laid the blame for this squarely on the industry, which 'has attracted large numbers of foreign workers without taking into account their living conditions, [...] and has left migrant workers living in the Afrikaander neighbourhood to fend for themselves'. The Dutch Communist party, represented by Ms De Vos-Krul, also took a fierce stand against the terms 'race riots' and 'racism' as used by the *Telegraaf* and *Televizier Magazine*, among others. In De Vos-Krul's view, it was not a matter of race but a matter of class, with 'businesses setting up some kind of modern slave trade without giving a thought to how these people should be housed'. Communist party member Mr Van der Meiden also spoke of a social conflict rather than a racial one 'against the Turks or any other kind of foreigner'. He believed that 'the more people are dependent on each other, the more conflicts will arise. To think that conflicts can be eradicated is not even an ideal anymore, it's a utopia'. In line with the other speakers, Liberal Democrat member Ms Schuiten-Wilmont avoided the word 'race' while searching for the cause of the riots in the council's failure to distribute residents evenly throughout the city. 'The Netherlands are full [...], Rotterdam is overcrowded and certain neighbourhoods of Rotterdam are bursting at the seams'.

Another remarkable difference between the media hysteria and the councillors' approach was that the latter did not side unconditionally with the foreign residents. On the contrary, Labour member Van der Have and Communist party member Van der Meiden spoke up for the Dutch residents, saying they found 'the forming of vigilante groups an entirely understandable and human response'. The Liberal Democrats also said they understood 'why some residents took matters into their own hands'. Alderman Jettinghoff pointed out the fear among the Dutch population of the 'high concentration of single foreign workers and foreign families'. When the socially charged term 'racial conflict' was finally uttered in the council meeting, it was Mayor Thomassen who used it rather than one of the councillors. In agreement with the *Telegraaf* and *Haagse Post* headlines, he stated that 'it is above all a conflict born out of alienation, which in this instance just happened to manifest itself as a difference between races. I just hope I will never have to hear some of the language used during the conflict again.' In his interpretation of the conflict he referred to the press release and police report issued on 15 August 1972, which states, among other things, that 'the police must crack down on the hooligans in order to restore the peace in the Afrikaander neighbourhood'.

The birth of the Rotterdam Act

The riots ultimately had lasting political consequences. After the violent conflicts, the council implemented a number of measures to get a better grip on the poor living conditions in working class neighbourhoods, which included subjecting landlords to stricter supervision and shutting down boarding houses. In the first months after the riots, almost three hundred Rotterdam boarding houses were closed. The proposal that caused the greatest outcry, however, was the distribution of non-Western foreigners throughout the city. It was to be the first attempt at a population distribution policy in the Netherlands. Several councillors agreed with Labour member Van Hattem that every effort needed to be made to avoid ghettoisation, and councillor Jettinghoff argued that special policies needed to be adopted to prevent future riots, such as the 'distribution of the foreigners or lowering their concentration'.

On 31 August 1972, the population distribution policy was extensively discussed by the city council, specifically a proposed decision by the mayor and aldermen concerning the housing of foreign workers, the so-called boarding house regulation. The discussion at the meeting centred on a passage of that decision, which states that 'an even distribution can be achieved by setting up a system of percentages specified per neighbourhood, redressing the balance between the number of housing permits issued to Dutch nationals, residents from other parts of the kingdom, and foreigners'. Labour member Van Hattem was first to take the floor. He stated that 'something is brewing in many parts of the city. It is not our task to fan the flames, but to restore peace to the neighbourhoods.' Communist Party member De Vos-Krul also found the proposed distribution by assigning percentages to neighbourhoods slightly disturbing:

> It reminds me of the situation in certain American neighbourhoods, which stipulate that the population must consist of 5% 'blacks' and 95% 'whites'. I realise that is not your intention, but we need to be careful that the idea doesn't take on a life of its own.

Liberal member Baggerman also held the view that by introducing a distribution policy based on regulating population percentages per neighbourhood, the council 'may well be entering extremely dangerous territory'.

Labour alderman Jettinghoff shared many of the objections raised and pointed out that discrimination based on ethnicity was illegal.

> People sticking together and forming groups for reassurance is an international phenomenon that has its origins in human nature itself, and is not down to the 'rottenness' of our society. It raises the question whether it is necessary to implement a population distribution measure that could expose us to accusations of deliberate discrimination. [...] In my opinion, introducing such measures would lead us down the path of discrimination. That is not acceptable.

His fellow alderman and Catholic People's Party member De Vos opposed Jettinghoff's point of view that the new system would constitute discrimination, pointing out that the majority of councillors were convinced that it would not. In his view, the real crux of the problem lay in the fact that there were too many boarding houses on too small a territory. He believed that this problem needed to be solved, and the quality of boarding houses improved, without resorting to the distribution of non-Western foreigners throughout the neighbourhoods. Ultimately, however, the clause was accepted by 21 votes to 13.

On 28 September 1972, the Rotterdam Council voted for the amended proposal that new Rotterdam residents be distributed across the city. In order to prevent jeopardising the demographic balance, a maximum of 5% of residents settling in the neighbourhood should come from another country, including Suriname and the Dutch Antilles. The percentage was chosen because these demographic groups made up almost 5% of the city's population. The council accepted this proposal by 25 votes to 10. The Rotterdam Act, as it was later called and which was also known as the 5% ruling, was born. In the same meeting, a fresh incident was also discussed. According to the police, residents of Slaghek Street in Hillesluis threatened to take action against a Turkish family that had obtained permission to settle there. On 1 March 1973, a year after the distribution proposal was accepted, Liberal member Koning again spoke out against the population distribution policy and suggested to revoke the 5% ruling. Koning pointed to 'the commotion sweeping the country and the overseas territories of the kingdom of the Netherlands, as well as the commotion within the European Community. [...] I am convinced that this regulation is discriminatory.' Koning's proposal was rejected by 27 votes against 14.

In 1974, the Council of State annulled the Rotterdam distribution policy on the grounds that it was in violation of articles 2 and 5 of the UN convention on the elimination of all forms of racial discrimination, which commits governments to eliminate discrimination and obliges them to guarantee the right to adequate housing irrespective of race. That does not mean that Rotterdam abandoned the idea of population distribution, however. On the contrary, the council continued to consider distribution an appropriate measure for reducing tensions in the old neighbourhoods, and as a means of stimulating the integration of newcomers and improving security. In the late 1970s, Rotterdam made another attempt to spread immigrants more evenly throughout the city, this time calling the process 'bundled deconcentration'. Policy memos such as *Leegloop en Toeloop* (Migration and Immigration) from 1979 emphasised the importance of improving the distribution of immigrants over the city, justifying its necessity as follows:

> There is no denying that unrestrained concentration leads to intolerance and aggression, and, by extension, discrimination. The original Dutch population is staying put while the increasing concentration exacerbates feelings of anxiety and insecurity, all of which leads to xenophobia. And what is more, it creates exactly that which we as Dutch people so often criticise about South Africa: apartheid!

The idea was to house as many foreign residents as possible in neighbourhoods whose population consisted of less than 16% immigrants. Catchphrases like 'well-balanced population structure' and 'prudent placement policies' were primarily aimed at concealing the integration arguments making this possible. The memo *Leegloop en Toeloop* puts it as follows:

> Urban dynamics are characterised by open encounters, that is to say, people meeting face to face in an atmosphere of mutual trust. To achieve this, people need to feel confident in their own culture and their own identity.

Migrants who experience such values in their own circles will enter our Western society with more confidence, more openness and less fear.

In protest against the city of Rotterdam's plans, various organisations started legal procedures against the council. While the judge dismissed their claim for repealing the policy, the parties managed to come to an agreement during the session to make an end to the Rotterdam policy of linking ethnicity to access to housing.

Strike three

In 2002, the Liveable Rotterdam party of the Dutch populist Pim Fortuyn won the Rotterdam municipal elections by a landslide. Coming out of nowhere, the party won 17 of the 45 seats in the traditionally Social Democratic City Council. The results shook Rotterdam politics to the core, and Liveable Rotterdam, as the largest party, formed a coalition with the Liberals and Christian Democrats. Under the guise of 'new politics', subjects like security and integration topped the political agenda, and the language at council meetings became coarser. If politicians had used emojis at the time, we would have been treated to a wide range of furious, flushed, hysterical faces. According to the new party, 'Islam' was the villain to blame for almost everything. Following Fortuyn's lead, who was quoted in De Volkskrant calling Islam a 'backward culture', the new city council organised Islam debates. The discussions revolved around whether hijabs should be worn in public, the construction of the Essalam Mosque in Hillesluis and the integration of Muslims in Rotterdam. The political debate became gradually fiercer, with ever more personal attacks and demonisation. Suggestions were made to institute an 'immigration stop' and to 'build a wall around Rotterdam' that would halt the influx of immigrants to the city once and for all.

For a long time, political conflicts in the city council had revolved primarily around socio-economic issues such as the distribution of wealth among citizens. In the 2000s, such conflicts gradually faded into the background to be replaced by a cultural conflict, which increasingly focused on identity, security, multiculturalism and how individuals related to the nation. In this vein, the city of Rotterdam made another effort to distribute immigrants in 2003, this time backed by the national government, the second Balkenende cabinet, after councillor of the borough of Charlois Dominic Schrijer raised the alarm that non-Western foreigners would make up almost half of the city's population by 2017. In Charlois itself, the proportion of foreign residents was even set to rise to 75%. The report Rotterdam zet door (Rotterdam Perseveres) from 2003, which was an indirect result of Schrijer's cry for help, states that 'colour is not the problem, but the problem is (often) coloured'. As a precaution to make sure the new proposal of introducing income requirements for residents looking to settle in certain neighbourhoods would be successful, and in order to defuse the situation politically as early as possible, the term 'foreign residents' was replaced by 'disadvantaged residents'. The report states:

> The absorptive capacity of certain neighbourhoods is exceeded by a continuous influx of disadvantaged residents while the privileged can afford to move to other parts of the city. We consider this, along with the resulting disturbances and illegal and criminal activities, to be at the heart of the problem.

The term 'disadvantaged residents', though central to the memorandum, is neither clearly defined nor elaborated anywhere – and given that the data concerns mainly Turkish, Moroccan, Surinamese, Antillean and Cape Verdean residents, it would in fact have been more accurate to speak of 'foreign residents'.

At the insistence of the city of Rotterdam, the second Balkenende government put forward a proposal for the Urban Areas Special Measures Act – also called the Rotterdam Act after its Rotterdam initiators – in 2004. The act was a nationwide implementation of measures taken by Rotterdam a year previously to halt the deterioration of disadvantaged neighbourhoods by imposing income require-ments on newcomers to the city. It enabled municipalities to apply for certain neighbourhoods to be designated as 'opportunity zones' if at least 45% of their residents had a low income and 25% no income from work at all. This meant than newcomers who had lived in the region for less than six years could be subjected to income requirements before being allowed to settle in the neighbourhood.

The proposal came under fire from the Council of State, the National Bureau against Racial Discrimination and the Equal Treatment Commission, who believed there was no objective justification for making the indirect dis-tinction arising from the new act between privileged and underprivileged Dutch citizens. And as the proposal mainly targeted new immigrants, it was also thought to lead to indirect racial discrimination. Neither the government nor the Rotterdam city council were swayed by the criticism, however, responding with the statement that there was in fact an objective justification: the fact that other, less far-reaching measures, had proved inadequate. They also rebutted the claim that it constituted direct discrimination, arguing that it was indirect racial or ethnic discrimination at most, which according to the alderman for physical infrastructure Marco Pastors of the Liveable Rotterdam party was justified by the act's purpose. 'Neighbourhoods that already present major problems now seem doomed to degenerate into ghettos. We must carry out this policy for the sake of the greater good.'

Since 2006, the Rotterdam Act has been implemented in the Rotterdam neighbourhoods of Hillesluis, Carnisse, Oud-Charlois, Tarwewijk and Bloemhof, all of which struggle with serious problems like vandalism, violence, burglary and drug use. Remarkably, a review of the Rotterdam Act has shown that the demographics in the designated neighbourhoods changed with the arrival of more middle-class residents and the decrease of residents on benefits, but that this has not increased liveability and security in those neighbourhoods, which have become no more safe or pleasant than before.[13] On the contrary, the neighbourhoods where the Rotterdam Act was implemented have deteriorated more than those where it was not, and are still considered problem areas.

Conclusion

Though the problems we face in modern times are hardly comparable with those of the past, hysteria about the arrival of asylum seekers and refugees is anything but a new phenomenon. Immigration hysteria rears its ugly head with great regularity, and when it does, people invariably pretend that society is on the brink of collapse. On 10 March 1994, during the war in former Yugoslavia (1994–2000), a *Telegraaf* headline announced there would be '100,000 asylum seekers this year', when in fact only 53,000 refugees applied for asylum in the Netherlands that year. Other recurrent experiences include arson, bomb scares and asylum centres being defaced with swastikas. People argued at the time that women were at risk from the men coming into the country; the number of refugees seeking asylum in the Netherlands doubled annually; Dutch culture would vanish if immigrants did not integrate; integration was achieved at the expense of 'ordinary Dutch people', as too much money was spent on asylum policies and immigrants; the government was not in control of the situation and unaware of the risks posed by the arrival of so many refugees; refugees were ungrateful for the time and money that society invested in them – precisely the same arguments that are bandied about today. In that respect, the current hysteria is not much different from past ones.

And yet we routinely dismiss hysteria about integration and immigration as a problem unique to today's world – a hysteria that stands in stark contrast to the fondly remembered atmosphere of solidarity and mutual trust in post-war Western countries, when no one locked their front door and neighbours walked in and out of each other's houses. The example of the Rotterdam race riots in the early 1970s clearly proves that the everyday problems we saw in the past are still presenting themselves today. This makes it difficult to form a final judgement on the way the media and politics reacted to the Afrikaander neighbourhood riots. One thing that is clear, is that they alternated between aversion and understanding. You could also say that hysteria constantly changes colour, or, as Wu-Tang Clan puts it in the song 'Gravel Pit', 'Back, back and forth and forth'. The press initially sided with the foreign population, focusing on the racist motives of the originally Dutch residents of the neighbourhood, and ignoring the underlying reasons for the erupting violence. Later research into the riots in the Afrikaander neighbourhood painted a subtler picture. While the rioters were by no means strangers to racism, there were many other issues at play, including housing shortage, rising unemployment, the deterioration of the neighbourhood and the feeling that the council was letting things slide while consistently ignoring the residents' complaints. Taken together, this goes a long way towards explaining the tension that gripped the neighbourhood.

The national media's hysterical hyperboles of war and Holocaust stood in marked contrast to the Rotterdam city council's initially calm, confident tone. Later, the council also changed its tune, especially in 2002, when the Liveable Rotterdam party 'was born and presented itself to the outside world with heated word games', to quote Peter Sloterdijk on the subject of hysteria.[14] What had originally revolved around poor housing conditions of foreign residents of the Afrikaander neighbourhood, gradually morphed into a completely different political frame – that of immigrants being the cause of misery in the old neighbourhoods, and its original residents their victims. From that moment on, the political debate hinged on the multicultural society and Islam. Race, culture and religion became decisive factors, and to top it off, the Rotterdam Act was implemented to curb the influx of foreigners into the city, leading to the exodus of those same residents to other neighbourhoods. It appears to be a case of what, in a different context, Canadian-American sociologist Erving Goffman called 'secondary gains',[15] as apart from posing a problem, the Afrikaanderwijk riots also seemed to offer the council certain advantages – it handed them an excuse to determine which residents were allowed to settle in which part of town.

Today, the Afrikaander neighbourhood has been eclipsed by the prestigious Kop op Zuid neighbourhood with its theatres, hotels, restaurants, cinema complexes, residential tower blocks, marinas and upmarket penthouses for white yuppies. The population of the South Rotterdam district, whose 200,000 inhabitants make it the seventh largest 'city' in the Netherlands, is still highly diverse and in a state of constant flux. Only Paarl Street no longer exists – by order of the mayor and aldermen, the name Paarl Street was revoked on 26 February 1988.

Notes

1 Sykes (2016).
2 The Afrikaander riots went down in history as the first race riots in the Netherlands, but in an article published in the *Historisch Genootschap Roterodamum*, historian Marlou Schrover points to riots that erupted in 1926 Rotterdam between Dutch seamen and foreign sailors, whom the papers called 'Arabs', 'darkies' or 'coloureds' without specifying their nationality. According to the papers, the riots broke out because Dutch sailors felt they were discriminated against – whenever one 'Arab' left his job, the vacancy would invariably be filled by another 'Arab'. *De Tijd* daily newspaper reported that the Dutch sailors feared this would create a 'great surplus of coloureds'.
3 Polderman (2007).
4 Cohen (1973, p. 62).
5 Verhoeven (2007, p. 62).

6 Goode & Ben-Yehuda (2009).
7 Cohen (1973, p. 61).
8 Becker (1963, p. 147 ff.).
9 Thompson & Williams (2014).
10 Cohen (1973, pp. 11, 162, 203).
11 Smelser (1962, p. 101).
12 Freud (2006d, p. 93).
13 Hochstenbach et al. (2015).
14 Sloterdijk (2003, p. 87).
15 Goffman (1968, p. 21).

Chapter 8

The success paradox

Hysteria is counted among the extinct mental disorders. Vanished from the GP's office, it has fallen through the cracks of medical history. Doctors and psychologists stopped diagnosing patients with hysteria after the condition was removed from the DSM, and the number of reported cases has plummeted to almost nothing as a result. This is remarkable, given that since time immemorial, hysteria has been considered an inherent source of misery in most people's lives. The condition, whose symptoms included palpitations, high blood pressure, indigestion and worse, was seen as a dreaded obstacle that prevented people from functioning normally. Often resulting in theatrical scenes, coarse language, an inner sense of loneliness, alienation, a loss of control and even of the will to live, hysteria has been a source of inspiration to many thinkers and scientists. No other illness has generated so much debate or proved such an inexhaustible source of scientific research. The condition has been the subject of a veritable flood of books with the word 'hysteria' in the title, and countless studies have been published that describe the causes and symptoms of hysteria in great detail. Some excellent books on hysteria include *Nervous, Hypochondriac or Hysteric Disorders* (1764), *The English Malady* (1773), *A Treatise on Hysteria* (1830) and *Hysteria and Certain Allied Conditions* (1897). Outbreaks of hysteria continued well into the twentieth century, and the frenzied scenes that accompanied them gave rise to countless books with such evocative titles as *Captain Dreyfus: The Story of a Mass Hysteria* (1955) and *Political Hysteria America* (1972).

It is reasonable to expect that with the disappearance of hysteria, the debate would subside and the illness would no longer be talked about, as happened in the cases of cholera, smallpox, leprosy and the plague – gruesome diseases which have all as good as disappeared and are hardly ever mentioned today. The opposite is true, however; hysteria never really went away. It is, on the contrary, a relatively stable element in – and a normal part of – human life. Hysteria is part of us, if not in the guise of an illness, then as a state of mind or a form of behaviour. For present-day manifestations of hysteria, you have to look no further than the consumer hysteria on Black Friday, to name one example. In this American phenomenon, which has spread to Europe in recent years, people storm the high street en masse in a frenzied hunt for bargains. They camp outside department stores until the doors open and they all squeeze in at once, trampling over each other, only to find that many of the bargains are not the deals they are cracked up to be – items are presented as special offers while their sales price is the same or even higher than it is elsewhere. You can also look at the hysterical housing market in London and New York, which has been completely disrupted by buyers being played off against each other and houses being sold for amounts well above the asking price. House prices being unprecedentedly high at the moment, it is only a matter of time until the hysteria will to come to a head and the housing market crash again. Other collective outbursts of violent emotions – bordering on hysteria – that appear in the media with some regularity include Bitcoin mania and the frenzied scenes surrounding any performance by South Korean boy bands, with shrieking, screaming, hyperventilating teenage girls fainting in droves.

Despite hysteria's exceptionally rich and extensively documented history, doctors, artists, philosophers and other scientists consistently fail to frame a simple answer to the mystery of hysteria. Views on the definition, symptoms, diagnosis and treatment of hysteria are as varied and even contradictory as the explanations of its cause, which range from a wandering womb to an Oedipus complex. If one thing is clear, it is that the psychoanalyst's perspective differs from that of the medical world, which in turn is very different from that of the philosopher. Everyone presents their own views from their own perspective. Some may focus predominantly on biological factors that make one person more prone to hysteria than another, while others highlight the subconscious processes conducive to the illness. An unwritten law seems to dictate that the more is known about hysteria, the more obscure it becomes, ultimately leaving it shrouded in mystery. For there is still no consensus on what exactly hysteria is – only that it exists.

For a long time, hysteria was surrounded by the most bizarre stories. No one nowadays would put the condition down to an anomalous blood flow from the womb to the brain, or claim sufferers were possessed by devils and demons. This leads to the conclusion that traditional explanations for hysteria are no longer valid and cannot in good faith be applied to present-day manifestations of hysteria. The condition is no longer described, for instance, in terms of subconscious, often sexually tinted, emotions and desires trying to find an outlet in bored upper-class women. This was thought to be caused by the Oedipus complex, in which a girl turns away from her mother in disappointment and is sexually attracted to her father. Thanks in a large part to the emancipation of women, this Freudian meaning of hysteria is no longer in use. As the American women's rights pioneer Charlotte Perkins Gilman wrote in *The Yellow Wallpaper* from 1892, society was sick, not female patients. It is true that Freud did not ignore the way the prevailing culture of his time oppressed women, but he limited his diagnosis to the suppression of sexual desires and fantasies. The women's movement, on the other hand, placed countless demands on the political agenda, ranging from female suffrage to the right to work. It would be wrong, however, to think that the women's movement achieving its aims led to the disappearance of inequality between men and women. Even today, the old prejudice that women are particularly prone to hysteria still exists; for example, male patients who are in pain after an operation are given painkillers, while female ones with the same complaints are prescribed sedatives.

Hysteria may no longer exist in a medical context, it is still ubiquitous in today's society. There are no hard statistics available, but hysteria seems to occur ever more frequently and have a greater impact on people's lives. Please note that I am not referring to the medical condition as anatomically and physiologically explained in the past as a hungry uterus (Plato) or a hereditary brain disease (Charcot). In the preceding chapters, I have discussed hysteria as a sociological phenomenon, focussing on the question why people get so wrought up about political moral issues such as liveability, security and immigration. Different though the three subjects are, they share a number of similarities when it comes to the high-running emotions they trigger and the conflicts they lead to. In the first place, all three subjects have become so large and complex as to go beyond the ordinary imagination of many citizens. Security, for example, cannot be defined in final terms, which makes it infinitely uncertain – there is, after all, no way of determining at which point we are completely safe. That is why citizens confronted with criminal behaviour in their neighbourhood either shut themselves off from it or fight back with excessive force. In the latter case, the feeling that they have lost control over their lives makes them cast themselves as victims, even if they have not actually been targeted by crime. Holding on to their victimhood, despite sometimes behaving aggressively towards others themselves, can lead to hysterical scenes. They have lost all sense of responsibility for their own behaviour and the way they express their emotions at this stage, to the point where they may actually lose control over their actions and have no clear memories of them later. An important factor in this is the need to be seen and heard – hysterical people scream for recognition, desperate for their situation to be acknowledged, and demand attention in the hope that people around them will take them seriously. In that respect, hysterical screams can be seen as a cry for meaning. This need for other people's attention, which can manifest itself in all kinds of ways, shows that hysteria is always also a collective issue. Another staple ingredient of hysteria is the violent expression of feelings and desires with the aim of making your voice heard. As a rule, hysterics make use of over-the-top language that is duly peppered with exclamation marks and capital letters and becomes increasingly formal over time. Citizens are fed this language through populism in politics and on social media. Anyone wanting to be heard in today's world needs to use words like 'unacceptable' and 'staggering'.

There are countless possible explanations for hysteria, though it would seem that the hysterical processes we are seeing now are largely being fuelled by the world around us. This means they are given meaning and direction by what the American philosopher Eugene Thacker called the 'world-for-us'.[1] Though we can know nothing about what the world is like in itself, we know a great deal about the world as we and our fellow humans experience it. This is the 'world-for-us' – the world as we perceive it and which we endow with meaning, the world we feel attracted to and from which we can become alienated. In my opinion, this relational aspect of hysteria is of great theoretical and practical importance for a better understanding of hysteria. If the history of hysteria has taught us anything, it is that the medical model, in which considerable importance is attached to an individual's autonomy, has dominated the analysis of hysteria to too great an extent. In this view, hysteria is considered a purely internal phenomenon that can be controlled with the correct diagnosis and appropriate medication, but the emphasis on autonomy and self-determination conceals the fact that we ourselves are an inherent part of the processes we reflect upon. We are constantly embedded, down to the capillaries of our nervous system, in assemblages of social and neurological relationships. The philosopher Henk Oosterling uses the term 'relational autonomy',[2] arguing that autonomy always occurs within the framework of a relationship. This seems to suggest that it can be informative to explore the link between hysteria and the society we live in today, as well as our physiological reaction to it, and the question which changes in society can cause certain emotions to arise and tip over into hysterical processes at a moment's notice.

Discussing hysteria, we tend to ignore the link between individual stories and the big picture, while hysteria has as much to do with the individual as with wider political, economic and cultural changes in society. Hysteria is unique in that it stems from internal processes that affect the nervous system, in contrast to such diseases as the plague, leprosy, cholera, typhus and TB, which come from the outside and infiltrate the body through microscopic bacteria or invisible viruses that spread through the air. But despite being a nervous disorder coming from within, hysteria is triggered by external stimuli. The philosopher Byung-Chul Han argues that we live in a neuronal era, in which we are threatened not so much by infections but a neuronal violence that leads to countless psychological infarcts. 'From a pathological standpoint,' Han writes, 'our century is determined neither by bacteria nor by viruses, but by neurons.'[3] Consequently, examining an individual's hysterical behaviour can tell us something about the society we live in. In this way, hysteria provides a key to the world we live in, as well as to a wide range of seemingly very diverse phenomena that all fall into the category of 'hysteria'.

The wider picture shows that hysteria is inextricably linked to the specific stage of the modernisation process we are in today. More than any other illness, it follows the movements of the changing organisational structure of society, and mirrors the culture of a certain period. This is clearly shown by the history of hysteria. In 1892, the Austrian physician and cultural pessimist Max Nordau wrote in his notorious book *Entartung* (Degeneration) that the growing number of cases of hysteria were down to the fact that people were unable to keep up with the rapid development of modern society. Comparing his analysis to a hellish tour through the hospital of the 19th century, he concludes that Western society is haunted by a '*schwarze Pest von Entartung und Hysterie*' ('black plague of degeneration and hysteria').[4] According to Nordau, hysteria is the result of exhaustion, which in turn is caused by the hectic lifestyle and excess of stimuli that characterise life in a large city. He describes an unhealthy fin-de-siècle feeling that was closely related to the way public life accelerated at the end of the 19th century – a time marked by technological changes following each other in quick succession, expanding the world and bringing with them a decreased sense of security. Age-old traditions and stories were pushed out by new media such as the telephone and the telegraph, which brought people together who had previously been far apart. Daily life was further intensified by the invention of the steam train, the gramophone and film, as well as the spectacular growth of cities, all of which brought people in touch with new sounds, images and worldviews. Everything that had once been small and familiar became large and overwhelming.[5]

Nordau's book gained notoriety for the way in which he reviles certain art movements he classes as 'mysticism'. According to Nordau, expressions of this 'degenerate art' are a sign of weakness and degeneration. While mainly targeting Symbolism and Impressionism, Nordau also pares down hysteria to an essential point, believing it is a bodily symptom of our conflict with the restless world-for-us, and the loss of security this makes us feel. In a time that saw the invention of the railway and the telephone, borders disappeared at a similar rate as in the current globalisation, driven by neoliberal thinking and social media. We are again seeing a steep decline of a primal sense of security, the social glue of society. This raises questions such as: Who am I, where do I belong, how important is my language, my culture, my history? In many countries, Anglo-Saxon neoliberalism has been replacing social democracy since the 1970s, leading to fewer borders and more anonymity. At the same time, the pillarisation of society made way for individualism, increasing people's vulnerability and loneliness and diminishing their influence. There has also been a marked decline of all kinds of social meeting places, ranging from public libraries and youth clubs to corner shops, which have disappeared or been replaced by corporations. Such places used to have a vital function in bringing people together and providing a sense of security, and this loss of security – often combined with feelings of fear, frustration and anger – is a recurrent factor in outbreaks of hysteria in our society. In that respect, life has arguably returned to how it was in late-19th-century Europe. Not that society is the same as it was at the time of Charcot and Freud, too much has changed since then, but there are undoubtedly some very striking similarities.

If the 21st century could lie on the analyst's couch, the first question to explore would be: What is making us hysterical? Is there a link between the constant outbursts of hysteria around such subjects as immigration, liveability and security? It seems to me that while such hysteria can be described in many different ways, it is undoubtedly fuelled by a culture that not only encourages and enjoys but also abuses and rewards it, through the media, the economy, and even in politics. These may seem like three very different spheres, but a look at their underlying structure reveals that they are not that far apart from each other. Hysteria has become their business model. Social media, which enable a much faster circulation of information – be it true or false – than in the past, both run on and produce hysteria. The danger of polarisation on social media is especially great when Facebook automatically places posts at the top of the timeline whose extreme outrage generate the most clicks, shares and comments, because they also bring in the most advertising revenue. This also goes for Twitter, which would go bankrupt tomorrow without hysteria.

The same is true for economy and politics, of which hysteria is an inherent part as well as a frequently used tool. By which I mean, they both make clever use of our desires. This may seem like a strange conclusion on the face of it, as both the economy and politics are considered fields in which calculated reason trumps messy human emotions – a view that is in line with the human ideal of the Enlightenment based on the rational and well-informed citizen striving only for the common good. But even if analyses of the economy and politics do not systematically use the term 'hysteria', they constantly draw on society's potential for hysteria. It goes without saying that this has a major impact on our emotional life.

One thing today's economy and politics have in common is the constant emphasis on a new void in our existence that cries out to be filled. Take politics. Many politicians seem to say, 'Give me a hysteria and I will give you hope', before promising a perfect society from which illness and crime have been completely eradicated. Every single political discussion about public safety, for instance, invariably leads to the unanimous conclusion that more decisiveness is needed to solve all problems for good. Once the diagnosis has been made, new rules and laws soon follow – only for the cycle to be repeated, time and again. Anyone suggesting that problems like this are too large and complex to be completely resolved or that it may be better not to act immediately, is irrevocably accused of 'looking the other way'. The economy also makes clever use of our existential fear of being socially inadequate. A customer buying a product today pays more for an idea or a brand than for the actual item, ostensibly because the idea or brand symbolises a certain experience. It is impossible to buy of a cup of coffee, a new phone or piece of clothing without the value of experience associated with them – in other words, without buying a whole lot more than the product. The experience economy, which is based on the premise that reality is the way people perceive it, expertly employs advertising and exposure to stimulate consumers' desires by creating a feeling of need in anyone who does not buy the latest mobile phone or sneakers.

Nothing is ever enough: four words that summarise today's ideology, in which our main drive is a constant feeling of need. This need, which psychoanalysts believe determines our identity to an important part, and which

Jacques Lacan calls a '*manque-à-être*' ('lack of being'), lies at the root of our desire. Just to be clear, this need does not precede that desire. We do not start out with an absence which then creates a desire in us to resolve our need. Need and desire are created simultaneously, making the desire self-generating. It perpetuates itself, because it both produces and is produced by itself. The desire does however involve a high degree of excessiveness, because no single object, experience or person can fully satisfy the need that lies at the root of the desire. As Mick Jagger put it, 'I can't get no satisfaction.' The desire, which can never be fulfilled, shifts continuously. Even if we obtain the thing we desire – which is all but impossible – it will only satisfy us temporarily. In fact, it makes no difference how we address the lack, as long as it helps us alleviate the frustration and impatience it causes.

It is interesting to approach this premise not only from a psychoanalytical perspective but to take a broader sociological view as well. How come we feel a lack when there is more than enough of everything in our society? What is the underlying reason for this? After all, we have never had it so good. We live in a time of unprecedented wealth and high levels of health care, and in a society that has never been safer. The list of top 10 happiest countries in the world is exclusively populated by Western countries, including Norway, Denmark, Canada and Australia. Our trust in each other is also rising, as is our trust in institutions such as the judiciary, the police force and the army. But that does not mean there is nothing wrong. Many people do not care about such rankings. Our inherent feeling of lack that has driven human development, bringing us wealth and progress, has also locked us in a stalemate and made us unhappy. For despite the fact we live longer, healthier and safer lives than our ancestors, many people feel that something is missing, and that feeling causes fear, frustration, anger and ultimately hysteria. The exact moment at which the former turn into the latter is difficult to pinpoint, but when hysteria is coupled with worry about things we care about, it cannot be underestimated or dismissed as benign – the calls for harsher punishment and revenge, the threats to mayors and aldermen and the hash tags with which all of this goes viral illustrate this. Hysteria may be dead to the medical world, the underlying mechanism in which pent-up feelings of fear, frustration and anger ultimately find an outlet in physical, hysterical reactions, is alive and well. This exposes a typical paradox of our time, which I would like to call the success paradox. The wealthier, healthier and safer our lives become, the more hysterical the last residue of lack makes us feel.

Hysteria is the world's revenge for reason. It invariably evokes a negative response and is seen as the greatest obstacle to human progress. Hysteria is used to accuse and dismiss others, who in turn denounce it as overly dramatic. 'Just be your normal self, that's crazy enough', as the Dutch saying goes. This suggests we have every reason to guard against hysteria. Writer Arnon Grunberg states, 'The real threat to the West are hysterical politicians and citizens.'[6] You often hear and read about the hysteria surrounding a certain subject being exposed. There, you see, it wasn't true – all that hysteria was unfounded.

Newspaper and television features such as Factcheck have made this their mission,[7] on the premise that hysteria is never constructive but only ever makes things worse. It never contributes to the solution of concrete problems. Hysteria does not compromise, it only polarises. That is why we cannot handle it.

Having said that, hysteria can also bring hope, in that it can galvanise people into action in the same way as a revolution can overthrow the establishment.[8] It has the power to turn the world upside down, just like the hysterical, uncontrolled laughter of the Joker in the eponymous film by director Todd Philips (2019) becomes a motto, a call to finish off today's rampant neoliberalism, after the Joker loses his medication and counselling because of budget cuts. Western history itself has shown that hysteria can lead to societal upheaval. A good example of this took place in the 19th century, when women started politicising their bodies to revolt against the suffocating conventions of the Victorian era. While hysteria led to many of its 'sufferers' being institutionalised, it also inspired social reforms aimed at giving women the same rights and opportunities as men. The tightly laced corset disappeared, making space for more liberal views on marriage, sexuality and the right to work. This is not hysteria in its most destructive, sinister form, in which people will tear off their clothes and pull out their hair – I am talking about a constructive hysteria which sets things in motion. Constructive hysteria is an engine for change, a way of making a contribution to the world. It acts for the greater good rather than out of self-interest.

Put simply, it seems to me that certain issues should be treated with a little less hysteria, while others could do with some more. The latter include illiteracy and poverty. Even societies where the average standard of living is high can contain groups of people who do not thrive. The Netherlands counts about 250,000 illiterate and one and a half million semi-literate people. Such figures do not make the headlines, you will not read about them in the paper. No one is raising the alarm over the fact that more than 4 million of the UK's 66.4 million inhabitants are trapped in deep poverty, including 2.3 million children. Nor does anyone seem too worried about a large part of this group being homeless and having to sleep in the open air or in covered public spaces such as railway stations and bicycle enclosures. There is no public outcry about this subject, and no one is working on a solution. Many politicians consider such matters distant problems, like dark clouds on the horizon that will eventually just blow over.

At the same time, eco-barbarism is running rampant. Entire libraries full of reports have been written in which the exact damage done by humans to the Earth is calculated. An 1800-page document published in 2019 by the UN environmental organisation IPBES, for example, shows that 75% of the Earth's land area and 66% of the oceans have been seriously damaged by human activity. Meanwhile, roughly 1,000,000 of the estimated 8 million plant and animal species on Earth are threatened with extinction, in many cases within a time frame ranging from a few years to a couple of decades. As journalist David

Wallace-Wells put it in his bestseller *The Uninhabitable Earth*, 'Here, the facts are hysterical.'[9] While the planet is hurtling towards its demise – an ocean with as much plastic in it as fish, rising sea levels and a steep decline of biodiversity – the debate focuses mainly on how much CO_2 we should be allowed to emit and what tax measures to take. We have turned a serious climate problem into a financial issue and made it our main goal to maintain the status quo. The debate about global warming invariably revolves around how much it will cost to go on living the way we are now, and includes painstaking calculations of exactly how much money needs to be spent on measures to preserve the planet as well as our lifestyles. This reduces an ecological issue to a bookkeeping problem, to be resolved by a flight tax here, an energy subsidy there. The real issue, that we need to develop a completely new ecological awareness as well as a new and more inclusive understanding of such matters as 'damage', 'care' and 'responsibility', is not addressed, while those are in fact urgent subjects that deserve more attention, and demand immediate action.

You could also say that their sheer scale and disastrous effects on society alone should justify a hysterical gesture. Silence and inaction are no longer options. We do, after all, live in a hysterical world – and we know it.

Notes

1 Thacker (2011).
2 Oosterling (2016).
3 Han (2015, p. 1).
4 Nordau (1892, p. 523).
5 At the end of the 19th century, doctors rejected the derogatory term 'hysteria' as a man's disease, preferring the term *neurasthenia*, which included similar symptoms such as nervous exhaustion, agitation, irritability and a general malaise. The neurologist George Beard, who popularised the term 'neurasthenia' with his book *A Practical Treatise on Nervous Exhaustion* from 1880, called neurasthenia a disorder of modernity, caused by the fast pace and pressures of urban life.
6 Grunberg (2015).
7 There has been a long tradition of trying to refute the facts that trigger mass hysteria in people, culminating in Charles Mackay's excellent 1841 book, *Extraordinary Popular Delusions and the Madness of Crowds*.
8 On resistance in contemporary social sciences, see: Hayward & Schuilenburg (2014) and Ferrell (2019).
9 Wallace-Wells (2019, p. 29).

Acknowledgements

My plan to write a book on hysteria for a broad audience was prompted by personal experience. On the occasions I am invited to speak on subjects like security on radio or national television, I often remark that we are in fact safer than politicians will have us believe. After such interviews, I invariably find dozens of angry e-mails in my inbox. 'Scandalous', 'Get a proper job', 'You're sucking up to the left-wing press' and 'Educate yourself' are among the least hostile comments I have received in recent years. Having said that, I did not write this book to prove a point – I take everyone seriously who looks up my contact details after a radio or television broadcast to vent their anger and frustration in an e-mail to me, and I always write a reply in which I try to explain my point of view. I am of course well aware that these are real complaints and concerns people have about such things as security and the current situation in the Netherlands. But I also believe it is vital to place these complaints and concerns in a wider sociological perspective, which is what I hope to have achieved in this book.

Hysteria is an adaptation of the original Dutch edition published by Boom Filosofie in 2019. This book differs from the Dutch version through extensive revision, updating and rewriting. The original version of *Hysteria* was written before the COVID-19 outbreak and the massive demonstrations against racist police brutality and systemic racism. As these events unfolded so rapidly, numerous updates and revisions kept postponing the translation of the final manuscript. In some cases, these revisions have been extensive, while in others only minor changes were deemed necessary. I hope that this has strengthened the book and made it more relevant to contemporary debates about issues such as security and immigration.

The English edition of this book would not have been possible without the help of friends and colleagues. I would like to thank Jeff Ferrell for writing such a fantastic foreword. I am grateful to Thomas Sutton of Routledge for his trust and support, and to Bob Hoogenboom, Barry Spunt, Rik Peeters and Ronald van Steden for their input and comments on various parts of the book. I would like to thank my translator Vivien Glass, who gave so much time and effort to translating the text into

English. The inspirational musical backdrop for writing this book was by Actress, Autechre, Sun Ra, John and Alice Coltrane, Morrissey, Lee 'Scratch' Perry and Sons of Kemet. Finally, I would like to thank my girlfriend, who regularly reminds me not to get stuck in my moods.

Movies and series

1984 (1956, Michael Anderson)
A Dangerous Method (2011, David Cronenberg)
A Scanner Darkly (2006, Richard Linklater)
Alien (1979, Ridley Scott)
Apocalypse Now (1979, Francis Ford Coppola)
Black Mirror (2016, season 3, Netflix)
Cape Fear (1991, Martin Scorsese)
Casino (1995, Martin Scorsese)
The Cleaners (2018, Hans Block & Moritz Riesewieck)
The Dark Knight (2008, Christopher Nolan)
The End of Violence (1997, Wim Wenders)
Equilibrium (2002, Kurt Wimmer)
Fahrenheit 451 (1966, François Truffaut)
Goodfellas (1990, Martin Scorsese)
Hysteria (2011, Tanya Wexler)
In the Mouth of Madness (1995, John Carpenter)
Invasion of the Body Snatchers (1956, Don Siegel)
Jagten (2012, Thomas Vinterberg)
Joker (2019, Todd Philips)
Leviathan (2014, Andrey Zvyagintsev)
Logan's Run (1976, Michael Anderson)
The Matrix (1999, Larry & Andy Wachowski)
Minority Report (2002, Steven Spielberg)
Predator (1987, John McTiernan)
Prince of Darkness (1987, John Carpenter)
The Purge (2013, James DeMonaco)
Raging Bull (1980, Martin Scorsese)
RoboCop (1987, Paul Verhoeven)
Silent Running (1972, Douglas Trumbull)
Soylent Green (1973, Richard Fleischer)
Strange Days (1995, Kathryn Bigelow)
Taxi Driver (1976, Martin Scorsese)

The Thing (1982, John Carpenter)
V for Vendetta (2005, James McTeigue)
The Walking Dead (2010, season 1, AMC)
WarGames (1983, John Badham)
The Wolf of Wall Street (2013, Martin Scorsese)
Z.P.G. (1972, Michael Campus)

References

Agamben, G. (1998). *Homo Sacer: Sovereign Power and Bare Life*. Stanford, CA: Stanford University Press.

Amnesty International (2013). *Proactief politieoptreden vormt risico voor mensenrechten: Etnisch profileren onderkennen en aanpakken*. Amsterdam: Amnesty International.

Balko, R. (2013). *Rise of the Warrior Cop: The Militarization of America's Police Forces*. New York: Public Affairs.

Bauman, Z. (1991). *Modernity and Ambivalence*. Cambridge: Polity Press.

Bauman, Z. (2000). *Liquid Modernity*. Cambridge: Polity Press.

Beccaria, C. (1963 [1764]). *On crimes and Punishments*. New York: Prentice-Hall.

Becker, H. (1963). *Outsiders: Studies in the Sociology of Deviance*. New York: Free Press.

Becking, B. (2015). *De Leviathan toen en nu: Afscheidscollege van de faculteit Geesteswetenschappen van de Universiteit Utrecht*. Utrecht: Universiteit Utrecht.

Beeckman, T. (ed.) (2009). *Spinoza: Filosoof van de Blijheid*. Brussels: ASP.

Bellow, S. (1964). *Herzog*. New York: Viking.

Benjamin, R. (2019). *Race after Technology: Abolitionist Tools for the New Jim Code*. Medford, MA: Polity Press.

Bent, E. van den (2010). Proeftuin Rotterdam: Bestuurlijke maakbaarheid tussen 1975 en 2005. Thesis, Erasmus Universiteit Rotterdam.

Berlin, I. (1969). *Four Essays on Liberty*. Oxford: Oxford University Press.

Bianchi, H. (1958). *Waar en waarom misdaad*. Amsterdam: Noordhollandsche Uitgeversmaatschappij.

Blokland, T.V. (2009). *Oog voor elkaar: Veiligheidsbeleving en sociale controle in de grote stad*. Amsterdam: Amsterdam University Press.

Bloom, P. (2016). *Against Empathy: The Case for Rational Compassion*. New York: HarperCollins.

Bolt, G. (2004). Over spreidingsbeleid en drijfzand. *Migrantenstudies*, 20(2), 60–73.

Bos, A. (1946). *De stad der toekomst, de toekomst der stad: Een stedebouwkundige en sociaal-culturele studie over de groeiende stadsgemeenschap*. Rotterdam: Voorhoeve.

Bowling, B., Parmar, A., & Phillips, C. (2011). Policing Ethnic Minority Communities. In T. Newburn (ed.), *Handbook of Policing* (pp. 611–641). London: Routledge.

Burroughs, W.S. (1959). *Naked Lunch*. New York: Grove Press.

Buuren, M. van (1991). Een barst waardoor het kwaad de ziel binnendringt: Hysterie en literatuur in de 19^e eeuw. *Revisor*, 18(6), 30–48.

Buuren, M. van, & Dohmen, J. (2013). *Van oude en nieuwe deugden: Levenskunst van Aristoteles tot Nussbaum*. Amsterdam: Ambo.

Çankaya, S. (2012). *De controle van marsmannetjes en ander schorriemorrie: Het beslissingsproces tijdens proactief politiewerk*. The Hague: Boom Lemma.

Carney, P., & Dadusc, D. (2014). Power and Servility: An Experiment in the Ethics of Security and Counter-Security. In M. Schuilenburg, R. van Steden & B. Oude Breuil (eds), *Positive Criminology: Reflections on Care, Belonging and Security* (pp. 71–84). The Hague: Eleven International Publishing.

Carr, P.J. (2005). *Clean Streets: Crime, Disorder and Social Control in a Chicago Neighborhood*. New York: New York University Press.

Cheyne G. (1733). *The English Malady: Or, a Treatise of Nervous Diseases of all Kinds, as Spleen, Vapours, Lowness of Spirits, Hypochondriacal, and Hysterical Distempers, etc.* London: Strahan.

Cixous, H. (1986). *The Newly-Born Woman*. Minneapolis, MN: University of Minnesota Press.

Cohen, S. (1973 [1972]). *Folk Devils and Moral Panics: The Creation of the Mods and Rockers*. St Albans: Paladin.

Das, A., & Schuilenburg, M. (2018). Predictive policing: Waarom bestrijding van criminaliteit op basis van algoritmen vraagt om aanpassing van het strafprocesrecht. *Strafblad: Tijdschrift voor wetenschap en praktijk*, 36(4), 19–26.

Dawkins, R. (1976). *The Selfish Gene*. Oxford: Oxford University Press.

Dekker, J., & Senstius, B. (2001). *De tafel van Spruit: Een multiculturele safari in Rotterdam*. Amsterdam: Mets & Schilt.

Deleuze, G. (1990). *Pourparlers 1972–1990*. Paris: Minuit.

Deleuze, G. (2004 [1968]). *Difference and Repetition*. London: Continuum.

Deleuze, G. (2005 [1981]). *Francis Bacon: The Logic of Sensation*. London: Continuum.

Devisch, I. (2017). *Het empathisch teveel: Op naar een werkbare onverschilligheid*. Amsterdam: De Bezige Bij.

De Waal, F. (1996). *Good Natured: The Origins of Right and Wrong in Humans and Other Animals*. Cambridge, MA: Harvard University Press.

De Waal, F. (2001). *The Ape and the Sushi Master: Cultural Reflections of a Primatologist*. New York: Basic Books.

De Waal, F. (2006). *Primates and Philosophers: How Morality Evolved*. Princeton, NJ: Princeton University Press.

De Waal, F. (2009). *The Age of Empathy: Nature's Lessons for a Kinder Society*. New York: Harmony.

De Waal, F. (2013). *The Bonobo and the Atheist: In Search of Humanism Among the Primates*. New York: Norton.

Didi-Huberman, G. (1982). *Invention de l'hystérie: Charcot et l'Iconographie photographique de la Salpêtrière*, Paris: Macula.

Dijksterhuis, E.J. (2000 [1950]). *De mechanisering van het wereldbeeld*. Amsterdam: Meulenhoff.

Douglas, M. (1966). *Purity and Danger: An Analysis of Concepts of Pollution and Taboo*. London: Routledge.

Draijer, N. (2008). Een razend verlangen naar betekenis: Over hysterie bij een borderline organisatie van de persoonlijkheid. In J. Dirkx & W. Heuves (eds), *Hysterie. Psychoanalytische beschouwingen* (pp. 83–99). Amsterdam: Boom.

Durkheim, É. (1960 [1893]). *De la division du travail social*. Paris: Presses Universitaires de France.

Eerden, P. van der (1994). De Malleus maleficarum, de duivel en de kwestie van de verdwenen geslachtsdelen. In G. Rooijakkers *et al.* (eds), *Duivelsbeelden: Een cultuurhistorische speurtocht door de Lage Landen* (pp. 137–167). Baarn: Ambo.

Elias, N. (2000 [1939]). *The Civilizing Process: Sociogenetic and Psychogenetic Investigations*. Oxford: Blackwell.

Engbersen, E., Snel, E., & Hart, M. 't (2015). *Mattheüs in de buurt: Over burgerparticipatie en ongelijkheid in steden*. Rotterdam: Kenniswerkplaats Leefbare Wijken.

Engelbrecht M. (2013). *De onttovering van de waanzin: Hoe het psychologische mensbeeld het magische verdrong (1550–1700)*. Amsterdam: Athenaeum–Polak & Van Gennep.

Eysink Smeets, M., Moors, H., Jans, M., & Schram, K. (2013). *De bijzondere belofte van Buurt Bestuurt: Maakt Buurt Bestuurt in de Rotterdamse praktijk de verwachtingen waar? En welke uitdagingen zijn er voor de toekomst?*Amsterdam: Lokaal Centraal.

Fabre, A. (1883). *L'hystérie viscérale: Nouveaux fragments de clinique médicale*. Paris: A. Delahaye & E. Lecrosnier.

Ferguson, A.G. (2017). *The Rise of Big Data Policing: Surveillance, Race, and the Future of Law Enforcement*. New York: NUY-Press.

Ferrell, J. (2019). In Defense of Resistance. *Critical Criminology*, 17 July. (doi: doi:10.1007/s10612-019-09456-6)

Foucault, M. (1978 [1976]). *The History of Sexuality, Volume I: An Introduction*. New York: Pantheon Books.

Foucault, M. (1989 [1963]). *The Birth of the Clinic: An Archeology of the Medical Perception*. London: Routledge.

Foucault, M. (2000). The Politics of Health in the Eighteenth Century. In J.D. Faubion (eds), *Michel Foucault: Power* (pp. 90–105). New York: The New Press.

Foucault, M. (2003). *Abnormal: Lectures at the Collège de France 1974–1975*. New York: Picador.

Foucault, M. (2006 [1961]). *History of Madness*. London: Routledge.

Freud, S. (2006a). *Werken 1, 1885–1899*. Amsterdam: Boom.

Freud, S. (2006b). *Werken 4, 1905–1909*. Amsterdam: Boom.

Freud, S. (2006c). *Werken 6, 1912–1915*. Amsterdam: Boom.

Freud, S. (2006d). *Werken 8, 1917–1923*. Amsterdam: Boom.

Freud, S. (2006e). *Werken 9, 1924–1929*. Amsterdam: Boom.

Galtung, J. (1969). Violence, Peace and Peace Research. *Journal of Peace Research*, 6(3), 167–191.

Garland, D. (2008). On the Concept of Moral Panic. *Crime, Media & Culture*, 4(1), 9–30.

Gemeentepolitie Rotterdam (1972). *Ongeregeldheden in Afrikaanderbuurt*. Rotterdam: Gemeentepolitie Rotterdam.

Gibson, W. (1984). *Neuromancer*. New York: Ace Books.

Gilman, C.P. (1892). The Yellow Wallpaper. *The New England Magazine*, January.

Gilson, F. (2010). Hysterie volgens Charcot: Opkomst en verdwijning van de 'zenuwaandoening van de eeuw'. Een medisch-historische studie. *Tijdschrift voor psychiatrie*, 52(12), 813–823.

Girard, R. (1988). *De zondebok*. Kampen: Kok Agora.

Goffman, E. (1968). *Stigma: Notes on the Management of Spoiled Identity*. London: Penguin.

Goldschmidt, W. (2006). *The Bridge to Humanity: How Affect Hunger Trumps the Selfish Gene*. Oxford: Oxford University Press.

Goode, E., & Ben-Yehuda, N. (1994). Moral Panics: Culture, Politics, and Social Construction. *Annual Review of Sociology*, 20, 149–171.

Goode, E., & Ben-Yehuda, N. (2009). *Moral Panics: The Social Construction of Deviance*. Oxford: Blackwell.

Gros, F. (2019). *The Security Principle: From Serenity to Regulation*. London: Verso.

Grunberg, A. (2015). Hysterie is de echte bedreiging. *De Volkskrant*, 19 November.

Hacking, I. (1986). Making Up People. In T. Heller, M. Sosna & D. Wellbery (eds), *Reconstructing Individualism: Autonomy, Individuality and the Self in Western Thought* (pp. 222–236). Stanford, CA: Stanford University Press.

Halasz, N. (1955). *Captain Dreyfus: The Story of a Mass Hysteria*. New York: Simon & Schuster.

Han, B.-C. (2015). *The Burnout Society*. Stanford, CA: Stanford University Press.

Harcourt, B.E. (2007). *Against Prediction: Profiling, Policing, and Punishing in an Actuarial Age*. Chicago, IL: Chicago University Press.

Harcourt, B.E. (2015). *Exposed: Desire and Disobedience in the Digital Age*. Cambridge, MA: Harvard University Press.

Harcourt, B.E. (2018). *The Counterrevolution: How Our Government Went to War Against Its Own Citizens*. New York: Basic Books.

Haute, P. van, & Geyskens, T. (2010). *De kunst van een onmogelijk genot: Klinische antropologie van de hysterie bij Freud en Lacan*. Utrecht: IJzer.

Hayward, K. & Schuilenburg, M. (2014). To Resist = to Create? Some Thoughts on the Concept of Resistance in Cultural Criminology. *Tijdschrift over Cultuur & Criminaliteit*, 4 (1), 22–36.

Hirschi, T. (1969). *Causes of Delinquency*. Berkeley, CA: University of California Press.

Hobbes, T. (1998 [1642]). *De Cive*. Cambridge: Cambridge University Press.

Hobbes, T. (2003 [1651]). *Leviathan*. Bristol: Thoemmes Continuum.

Hochstenbach, C., Uitermark, J., & Gent, W. van (2015). *Evaluatie effecten Wet bijzondere maatregelen grootstedelijke problematiek ('Rotterdamwet') in Rotterdam*. Amsterdam: Universiteit van Amsterdam.

Hume, D. (2011). *The Essential Philosophical Works*. Ware: Wordsworth.

Jentsch, E.A. (1995 [1906]). Zur Psychologie des Unheimlichen / On the Psychology of the Uncanny (trans. R. Sellars). *Angelaki: Journal of the Theoretical Humanities*, 2, 7–16.

Klinenberg, E. (2018). *Palaces for the People: How Social Infrastructure Can Help Fight Inequality, Polarization, and the Decline of Civic Life*. New York: Broadway Books.

Koehler, P.J. (1995). Freud, Charcot en de neurologische visie op hysterie. *Nederlands Tijdschrift Geneeskunde*, 139(43), 2177–2183.

Krznaric, R. (2014). *Empathy: Why it Matters, and How to Get It*. London: Random House.

Lacan, J. (1964). *Les quatre concepts fondamentaux de la psychanalyse*. Paris: Seuil.

Land, M. van der, & Stokkom, B. van (2015). Burgerparticipatie en 'crafting' in het lokale veiligheidsbeleid. *Tijdschrift voor Veiligheid*, 14(1), 3–21.

Landman, W., & Kleijer-Kool, L. (2016). *Boeven vangen: Een onderzoek naar proactief politieoptreden*. Amersfoort: Politie & Wetenschap.

Landouzy, H. (1846). *Traité complet de l'hystérie*. Paris: Baillière.

Lasch, C. (1980). *The Culture of Narcissism: American Life in an Age of Diminishing Expectations*. London: Sphere Books.

Levin, M.B. (1972). *Political Hysteria in America: The Democratic Capacity for Repression*. New York: Basic Books.

Locke, J. (2015 [1689]). *Second Treatise of Civil Government*. Claremont: Broadview Press.

Lombroso, C. (2006 [1876]). *Criminal Man*. Durham, NC: Duke University Press.

Luhmann, N. (2000). Familiarity, Confidence, Trust: Problems and Alternatives. In D. Gambetta (eds), *Trust: Making and Breaking Cooperative Relations* (pp. 94–107). Oxford: Department of Sociology, University of Oxford.

Mackay, C. (2003 [1841]). *Extraordinary Popular Delusions and the Madness of Crowds*. Petersfield: Harriman House.

Martelaere, P. de (2003 [1993]). *Een verlangen naar ontroostbaarheid: Over leven, kunst en dood*. Amsterdam: Aula.

Mauss, M. (2002 [1923–1924]). *The Gift: The Form and Reason for Exchange in Archaic Societies*. London: Routledge.

McGarry, R. & Walklate, S. (2019). *A Criminology of War*. Bristol: Bristol University Press.

McSweeney, B. (1999). *Security, Identity, and Interests: A Sociology of International Relations*. Cambridge: Cambridge University Press.

Micale, M.S. (2008). *Hysterical Men: The Hidden History of Male Nervous Illness*. Cambridge, MA: Harvard University Press.

Mooij, A. (1987 [1975]). *Taal en verlangen. Lacans theorie van de psychoanalyse*. Meppel: Boom.

Morgan, T. (2012). *Literary Outlaw: The Life and Times of William S. Burroughs*. New York: Norton.

Mutsaers, P. (2013). A Public Anthropology of Policing: Law Enforcement and Migrants in the Netherlands. Thesis, Tilburg University.

Neocleous, M. (2019). Securitati Perpetuae: Death, Fear and the History of Insecurity. *Radical Philosophy*, 2.06.

Netherlands Police Institute (2005). *Politie in ontwikkeling: Visie op de politiefunctie*. The Hague: NPI.

Netherlands Scientific Council for Government Policy (2016). *Big Data in a Free and Secure Society*. Amsterdam: Amsterdam University Press.

Nordau, M. (1892). *Entartung*. Berlin: Duncker.

Oosterling, H. (2013). *ECO3: Doendenken*. Heijningen: Japsam Books.

Oosterling, H. (2016). *Waar geen wil is, is een weg: Doendenken tussen Europa en Japan*. Amsterdam: Boom.

Pankejeff, S. (1972). My Recollections of Sigmund Freud. In M. Gardiner (ed.), *The Wolf-Man and Sigmund Freud*. London: Hogarth.

Peeters, R., & Drosterij, G. (2011). Verantwoordelijke vrijheid: Responsabilisering van burgers op voorwaarden van de staat. *Tijdschrift voor beleid, politiek en maatschappij*, 38(2), 179–199.

Peeters, R., & Schuilenburg, M. (2018). Machine Justice: Governing Security through the Bureaucracy of Algorithms. *Information Polity: An International Journal of Government and Democracy in the Information Age*, 23(3), 267–280.

Pierotti, R., & Fogg, B.R. (2017). *The First Domestication: How Wolves and Humans Coevolved*. New Haven, CT: Yale University Press.

Pinker, S. (2011). *The Better Angels of Our Nature: A History of Violence and Humanity*. London: Penguin.

Plato (2013 [c.360 BCE]). *Timaeus and Critias* (trans. A.E. Taylor). London: Routledge.

Plato (2015 [c.380 BCE]). *The Republic*. Irvine, CA: Xist.

Plautus (2006 [2nd century BCE]). *Asinaria: The One about the Asses* (trans. J. Henderson). Madison, WI: University of Wisconsin Press.

Polderman, C. (2007). 'Deze nood breekt elke wet': Het antwoord van de lokale politiek op de Rotterdamse Turkenrellen van 1972. *Holland, Historisch Tijdschrift*, 39(4), 257–275.

Preston, G.H. (1897). *Hysteria and Certain Allied Conditions*. Philadelphia, PA: Blakiston.

Putnam, R. (2000). *Bowling Alone: The Collapse and Revival of American Community*. New York: Simon & Schuster.

Ricard, M. (2015). *Altruism: The Science and Psychology of Kindness*. London: Atlantic Books.

Rousseau, J. (2003 [1755]). *Vertoog over de ongelijkheid*. Amsterdam: Boom.

Sampson, R.J., & Raudenbush, S.W. (2004). Seeing Disorder: Neighborhood Stigma and the Social Construction of 'Broken Windows'. *Social Psychology Quarterly*, 67(4), 319–342.

Sampson, R.J., Raudenbush, S.W., & Earls, F. (1997). Neighborhoods and Violent Crime: A Multilevel Study of Collective Efficacy. *Science*, 277(5328), 918–924.

Saunders, D. (2012). *Arrival City: How the Largest Migration in History is Reshaping Our World*. New York: Vintage Books.

Schermers, D. (1906). Eenige statistische beschouwingen over de psychosen in de Nederlandsche krankzinnigengestichten gedurende de jaren 1875–1900. *Psychiatrische en Neurologische Bladen*, 10, 39–42.

Schrover, M. (2012). Van zeeliedenoproer tot 'Pogrommerdam'. *Historisch Genootschap Roterodamum*, 1(3), 18–23.

Schuilenburg, M. (2015a). Behave or Be Banned? Banning Orders and Selective Exclusion from Public Space. *Crime, Law and Social Change*, 64(4–5), 277–289.

Schuilenburg, M. (2015b). *The Securitization of Society: Crime, Risk, and Social Order*. New York: New York University Press.

Schuilenburg, M. (2016). Predictive Policing: De opkomst van een gedachtenpolitie? *Ars Aequi*, 65(12), 931–936.

Schuilenburg, M., & Peeters, R. (2017). Gift Politics: Exposure and Surveillance in the Anthropocene. *Crime, Law and Social Change*, 68(5), 563–578.

Schuilenburg, M., & Steden, R. van (2014). Positive Security: A Theoretical Framework. In M. Schuilenburg, R. van Steden & B. Oude Breuil (eds), *Positive Criminology: Reflections on Care, Belonging and Security* (pp. 19–32). The Hague: Eleven International Publishing.

Schopenhauer, A. (1844 [1818]). *Die Welt als Wille und Vorstellung*, vol. 2. Leipzig: Brockhaus.

Scull, A. (2009). *The Disturbing History of Hysteria*. Oxford: Oxford University Press.

Seligman, M.E.P, & Csikszentmihalyi, M. (2000). Positive Psychology: An Introduction. *American Psychologist*, 55(1), 5–14.

Sennett, R. (2012). *Together: The Rituals, Pleasures and Politics of Cooperation*. London: Allen Lane.

Showalter E. (1997). *Hystories: Hysterical Epidemics and Modern Culture*. London: Picador.

Skogan, W.G. (2006). *Police and Community in Chicago: A Tale of Three Cities*. Oxford: Oxford University Press.

Sloterdijk, P. (2003 [1998]). *Sferen: Bellen & globes*. Amsterdam: Boom.

Sloterdijk, P. (2009 [2004]). *Sferen: Schuim*. Amsterdam: Boom.

Smelser, N.J. (1962). *Theory of Collective Behavior*. London: Routledge & Kegan Paul.

Sontag, S. (1990). *Illness as Metaphor and AIDS and Its Metaphors*. New York: Picador.

Stokkom, B. van, & Toenders, N. (2010). *De sociale cohesie voorbij: Actieve burgers in ach-terstandswijken*. Amsterdam: Pallas.

Stokkom, B. van, Eikenaar, T., & Becker, M. (2012). *Participatie en vertegenwoordiging: Burgers als trustees*. Amsterdam: Amsterdam University Press.

Stuart S. (2011). War as Metaphor and the Rule of Law in Crisis: The Lessons We Should Have Learned from the War on Drugs. *Southern Illinois University Law Journal*, 36(1), 1–43.

Sykes, C. (2016). Charlie Sykes on Where the Right Went Wrong. *The New York Times*, 15 December.

Tarde, G. (1969 [1901]). The Public and the Crowd. In G. Tarde, *On Communication and Social Influence* (ed. T.N. Clark) (pp. 277–294). Chicago, IL: University of Chicago Press.

Tate, G. (1830). *A Treatise on Hysteria*. London: Highley.

Taylor, C. (1979). What's Wrong with Negative Liberty? In A. Ryan (ed.), *The Idea of Freedom* (pp. 175–193). London: Oxford University Press.

Thacker, E. (2011). *In the Dust of This Planet. Horror of Philosophy*, vol. 1. Winchester: Zero Books.

Thompson, B., & Williams, A. (2014). *The Myth of Moral Panic: Seks, Snuff, and Satan*. New York: Routledge.

Tonkens, E. (2009). *Tussen onderschatten en overvragen: Actief burgerschap en activerende organisaties in de wijk*. Amsterdam: SUN.

Trillat, E. (1986). *Histoire de l'hystérie*. Paris: Seghers.

Tyler, T. (2001). Public Trust and Confidence in Legal Authorities: What Do Majority and Minority Group Members Want from the Law and Legal Institutions? *Behavioral Sciences and the Law*, 19, 215–235.

UNDP (1994). *Human Development Report: New Dimensions of Human Security*. New York: UNDP.

United Nations (2003). *Human Security – Now: Report of the Commission on Human Security*. New York: Verenigde Naties.

Veith, I. (1965). *Hysteria: The History of a Disease*. Chicago, IL: University of Chicago Press.

Verhaeghe, P. (1996). *Tussen hysterie en vrouw: Van Freud tot Lacan: een weg door honderd jaar psychoanalyse*. Leuven: Acco.

Verhaeghe, P. (1997). Trauma en hysterie bij Freud en Lacan. *Tijdschrift voor Psychoanalyse*, 2, 86–99.

Verhoeven, C. (2007 [1967]). *Inleiding tot de verwondering*. Utrecht: Ambo.

Vitale, A.S. (2017). *The End of Policing*. London: Verso.

Wallace-Wells, D. (2019). *The Uninhabitable Earth: Life After Warming*. New York: Tim Duggan Books.

Weber, M. (2006 [1904/1905]). *Die protestantische Ethik und der Geist des Kapitalismus*. Munich: Beck.

Weber, M. (2006 [1921/1922]). *Wirtschaft und Gesellschaft*. Paderborn: Voltmedia.

Webster, R. (1995). *Why Freud was Wrong: Sin, Science and Psychoanalysis*. New York: Basic Books.

Whytt, R. (1764). *Observations on the Nature, Causes, and Cure of Those Disorders which Have Been Commonly Called Nervous, Hypochondriac, or Hysteric: To which Are Prefixed Some Remarks on the Sympathy of the Nerves*. Edinburgh: Becket, DeHondt, and Balfour.

Willems, D., & Doeleman, R. (2014). Predictive Policing – wens of werkelijkheid? *Tijdschrift voor de Politie*, 76(4/5), 39–42.

Wilson, J.Q. (1985). *Thinking About Crime*. New York: Vintage.

Wilson, J.Q., & Kelling, G. (1982). Broken Windows. *Atlantic Monthly*, 249(3), 29–38.

Woolsey, R.M. (1976). Hysteria: 1875 to 1975. *Diseases of the Nervous System*, 37(7), 379–386.

Young, J. (2009). Moral Panic: Its Origins in Resistance, Ressentiment and the Translation of Fantasy into Reality. *British Journal of Criminology*, 49(1), 1–3.

Young, J. (2011). Moral Panics and the Transgressive Other. *Crime, Media, Culture*, 7(3), 245–258.

Zedner, L. (2007). Pre-crime and Post-criminology. *Theoretical Criminology*, 11(2), 261–281.

Zimring, F. (2012). *The City that Became Safe*. Oxford: Oxford University Press.

Zuboff, S. (2019). *The Age of Surveillance Capitalism. The Fight for a Human Future at the New Frontier of Power*. London: Profile Books.

Index

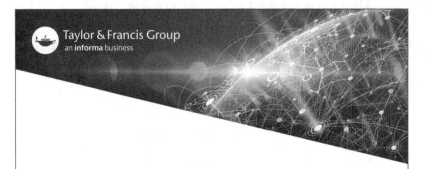